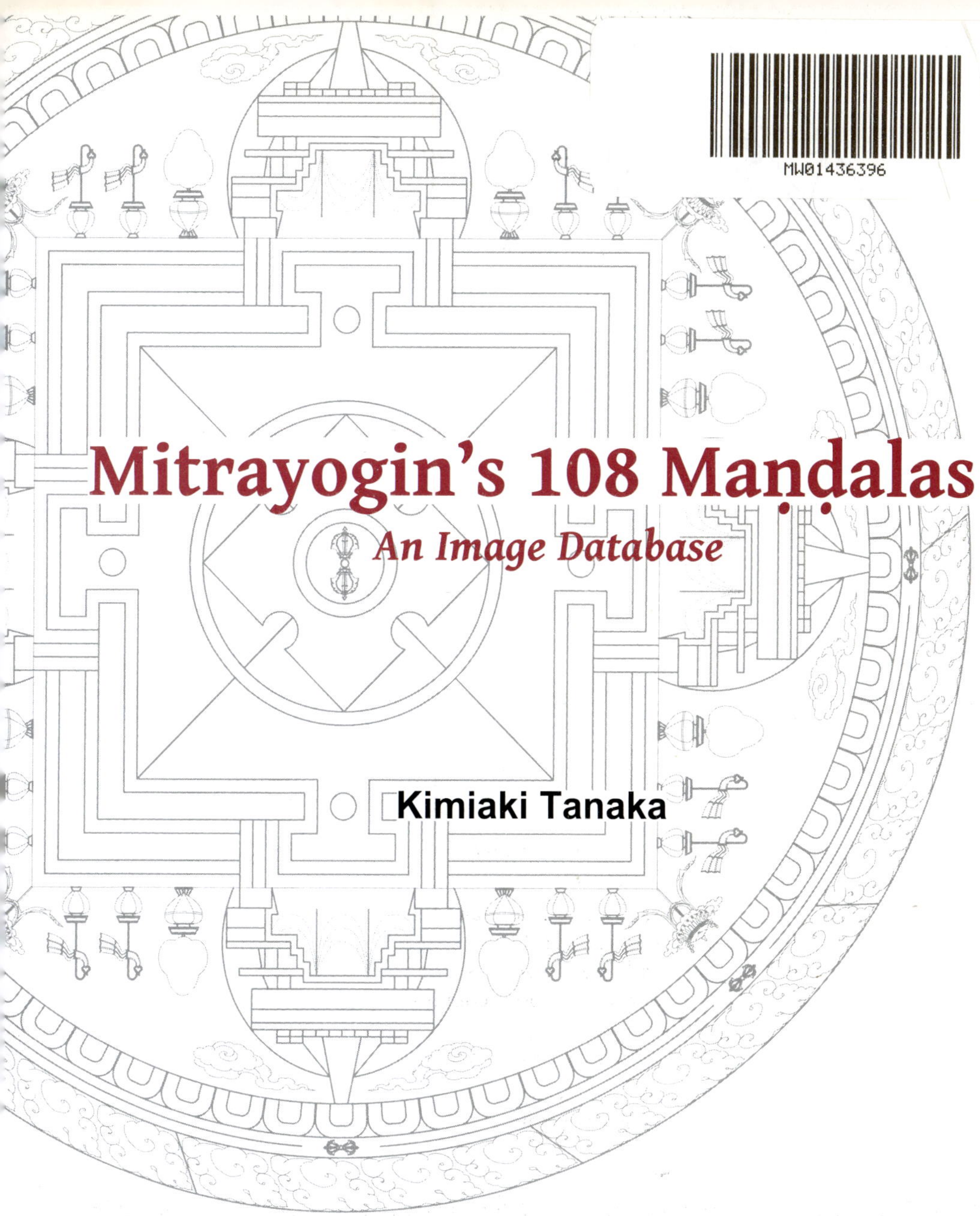

Mitrayogin's 108 Maṇḍalas

An Image Database

Kimiaki Tanaka

Vajra Publications
www.vajrabooks.com.np

Published by

Vajra Publications
Jyatha, Thamel, Kathmandu, Nepal
Tel.: 977-1-4220562, Fax: 977-1-4246536
e-mail: bidur_la@mos.com.np
www.vajrabooks.com.np

Distributed by

Vajra Books
Kathmandu, Nepal

ISBN No. 978-9937-506-92-2

Layout by Nabindra Dongol

Printed in Nepal

Contents

Legend ... 3

Mitrayogin's Collection of One Hundred Maṇḍalas and Their Iconography: The Handscrolls Held by the Hahn Cultural Foundation ... 5

Colour Schemes of the Courtyard ... 14

Explanatory Remarks on the *Vajrāvalī* Set of Maṇḍalas ... 17
- Highest Yoga Tantras ... 18
- Yoga Tantras ... 54
- Caryā Tantras ... 57
- Kriyā Tantras ... 58

Explanatory Remarks on the *Mitra brgya rtsa* Set of Maṇḍalas ... 63
- Kriyā Tantras ... 64
- Caryā Tantras ... 85
- Yoga Tantras ... 86
- Highest Yoga Tantras ... 104

Selected Bibliography ... 129

Index of Maṇḍalas ... 130

On the Hahn Cultural Foundation, Seoul ... 133

Toga Meditation Museum and Tibet Culture Centre International ... 135

Legend

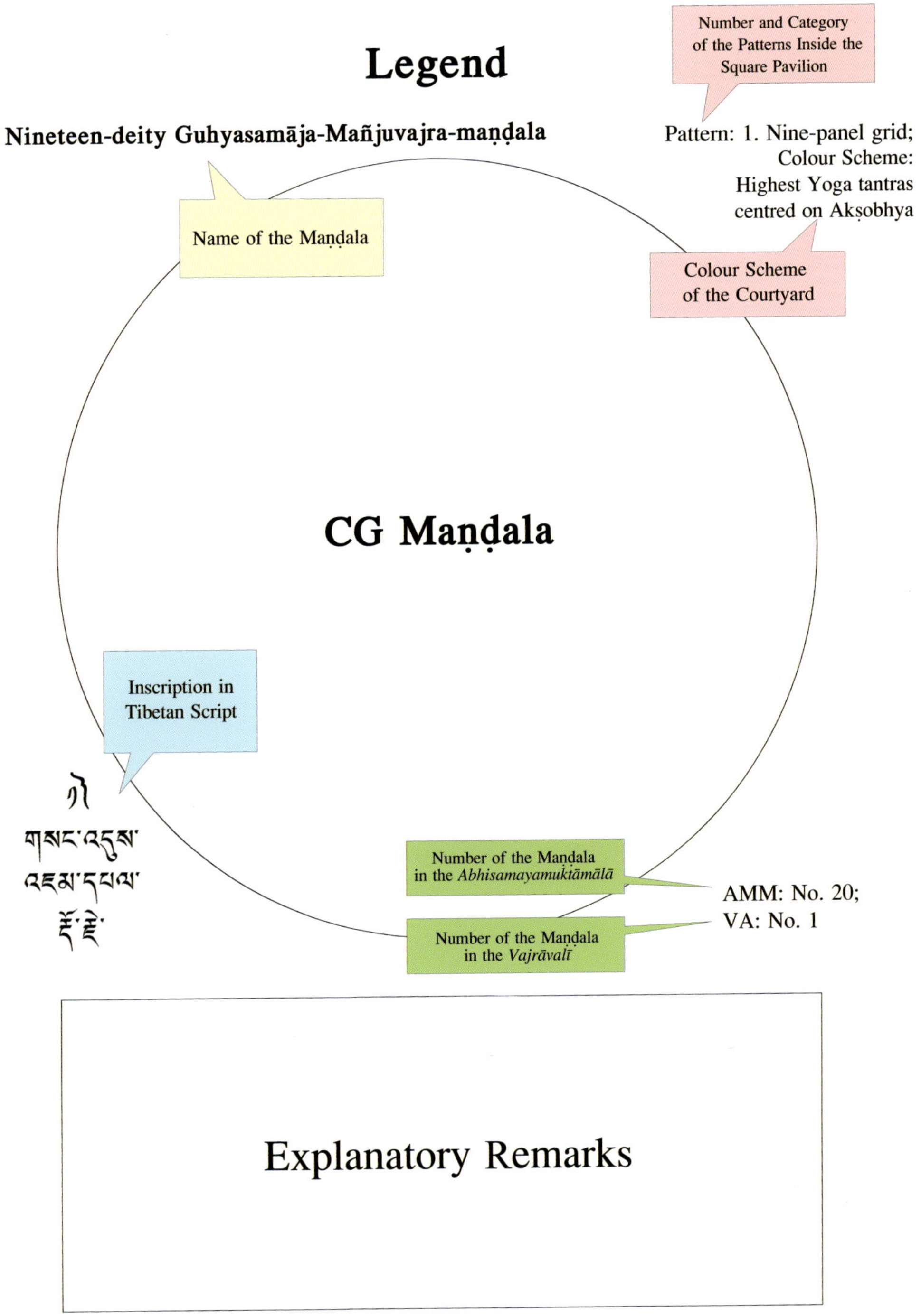

Number and Category of the Patterns Inside the Square Pavilion
Nineteen-deity Guhyasamāja-Mañjuvajra-maṇḍala
Pattern: 1. Nine-panel grid; Colour Scheme: Highest Yoga tantras centred on Akṣobhya
Name of the Maṇḍala
Colour Scheme of the Courtyard
CG Maṇḍala
Inscription in Tibetan Script
ཀ།
གསང་འདུས་
འཇམ་དཔལ་
རྡོ་རྗེ་
Number of the Maṇḍala in the *Abhisamayamuktāmālā*
AMM: No. 20; VA: No. 1
Number of the Maṇḍala in the *Vajrāvalī*
Explanatory Remarks

Mitrayogin's Collection of One Hundred Maṇḍalas and Their Iconography: The Handscrolls Held by the Hahn Cultural Foundation

Introduction

In the late twelfth century, when Indian Buddhism was on the brink of annihilation as a result of repeated Muslim invasions, Mitrayogin, an Indian Tantric adept who had taken refuge in the Kathmandu Valley in Nepal, received an invitation from the Tibetan translator Khro phu lo tsā ba (1173–1225) to visit Tibet, and in 1198–99 he resided in Khro phu monastery in gTsang, Tibet, where he transmitted the entire repertoire of maṇḍalas with which he was familiar. The 108 maṇḍalas transmitted by Mitrayogin on this occasion are known in Tibet as "Mitra's One Hundred" (*Mitra brgya rtsa*). Indian Buddhism disappeared soon after his visit to Tibet, and so these maṇḍalas became a precious heritage which represents the final stage in the 700-year development of the maṇḍala in India.

Later, the *Mitra brgya rtsa* was combined in Tibet with another maṇḍala set, the *Vajrāvalī* by Abhayākaragupta (1064-1125?), and together these came to be known as the "*Vajrāvalī* and *Mitra*" (*rDor phreṅ daṅ Mitra*). Most of the forty-two maṇḍalas explained in the *Vajrāvalī* are also included in the *Mitra brgya rtsa*, and this would seem to be why these two traditions were later merged into one system in Tibet. This tradition has continued down to modern times, and according to one account, in 1938 a high priest from bKra shis lhun po (Tashilhunpo) monastery, Ṅag chen dar ba Hu thug thu (1884–1947), conferred an initiation into these maṇḍalas on a total of 548 monks and laymen who had gathered from inland China, Mongolia and Tibet. The iconographical compendium entitled *Mitra daṅ rdor phreṅ gi lha tshogs kyi gtso bo'i sku brñan mthoṅ ba don ldan* (Delhi, 1985) is a reproduction of the Beijing lithograph edition published at Fazangsi 法藏寺 in Beijing on the occasion of this initiation rite (hereafter referred to as the Fazangsi lithograph).

The Handscrolls Held by the Hahn Cultural Foundation

Several collections of depictions of the main deities of the *Mitra brgya rtsa* are known to have existed in Tibet, but the existence of a complete maṇḍala set of the *Mitra brgya rtsa* had until recently not been reported.

However, in a Japanese collection that I was asked to appraise in 1991, I found a collection of maṇḍalas in the form of two handscrolls 46 × 540 cm and 46 × 800 cm in size, and I discovered that they represented complete sets of the *Vajrāvalī* and *Mitra brgya rtsa*. There is an inscription at the end that reads: "These are all the maṇḍalas of Maitri, and in addition there are also the Sixteen Drops and Antarsādhana-Amitāyus (*Mai tri'i dkyil 'khor cha tshaṅ yod / gzhan yaṅ thig le bcu drug tshe dpag naṅ sgrub yod*)." "Maṇḍalas of Maitri" is an error for "maṇḍalas of Mitra," and upon closer investigation I discovered that these two handscrolls constitute a complete set of Mitrayogin's collection of one hundred maṇḍalas.

Subsequently, these scrolls were purchased by the Hahn Cultural Foundation in Korea and were included in Vol. 2 of their official catalogue, *Art of Thangka* (Seoul, 1999). In 2001 they were exhibited at five museums in Japan during "The World of Thangka" exhibition and also at the "Tibetan Legacy" exhibition in 2003 at the British Museum. (These scrolls are hereafter referred as the "Hahn Foundation handscrolls.")

Textual Sources and Iconometry

In 1988, I purchased a book on the iconometry of the *Vajrāvalī* and *Mitra brgya rtsa*, *rDor phreṅ daṅ mitra sogs dkyil chog rnam las 'byuṅ ba'i yi dam rgyud sde bźi yi dkyil 'khor so so'i naṅ thig mi 'dra ba'i khyad par bśad pa, bso rig mdzes pa'i kha rgyan* (Delhi 1978; hereafter referred to as *Roṅ tha's Iconometry*) by Roṅ tha Blo bzaṅ dam chos rgya mtsho (1865–?), and came to know of the existence of these maṇḍala sets. But I was unable to undertake a detailed study since I did not know their textual source and did not have any example of a set of the *Mitra brgya rtsa*.

Professor Masahide Mori of Kanazawa University, meanwhile, discovered that the *Abhisamayamuktāmālā* (Peking No. 5022) and *Patraratnamālā* (Peking No. 5021) by Mitrayogin represent the textual sources of the *Mitra brgya rtsa*. The *Abhisamayamuktāmālā* explains the iconography, arrangement and visualization of the deities, while the *Patraratnamālā* provides a summary of the names of the 108 maṇḍalas and the number of deities of each maṇḍala. However, Professor Mori was unable to study the iconometry and design of the maṇḍalas that are not explained in the *Abhisamayamuktāmālā* and *Patraratnamālā* since the existence of the Hahn Foundation handscrolls was not yet known.

If we compare Professor Mori's study, the Hahn Foundation handscrolls, and *Roṅ tha's Iconometry*, we can reach a clear understanding of the iconometry, design and colour scheme of each maṇḍala. In this way, the Hahn Foundation handscrolls are very important for the study of the Tibetan maṇḍala.

The Hahn Foundation Handscrolls

Next, I wish to survey the contents of the Hahn Foundation handscrolls. The *Abhisamayamuktāmālā* explains 108 maṇḍalas in total. The Hahn Foundation handscrolls, on the other hand, depict forty-five maṇḍalas in the *Vajrāvalī* and sixty-five in the *Mitra brgya rtsa*. (Hereafter abbreviations will be used to refer to maṇḍalas in these two sets. For example, V-1 signifies the first maṇḍala of the *Vajrāvalī*, while M-3 signifies the third maṇḍala of the *Mitra brgya rtsa*.)

We can detect a slight difference in style between the two handscrolls. But in view of the fact that the *Mitra brgya rtsa* duplicates none of the maṇḍalas found in the *Vajrāvalī* collection, there is a strong possibility that the maṇḍalas from the *Vajrāvalī* included in the *Mitra brgya rtsa* were deliberately omitted in the handscroll of the latter. This would suggest that these two maṇḍala collections in handscroll format originally formed a set.

If we tally the number of maṇḍalas depicted in the two handscrolls, they come to 110. This number does not coincide with the 108 mentioned in the *Abhisamayamuktāmālā*. The comment in the inscription, namely, that "these are all the maṇḍalas of Maitri, and in addition there are also the Sixteen Drops and Antarsādhana-Amitāyus," would seem to explain the reason that the total number of maṇḍalas is not 108 but 110. But strangely the maṇḍalas of the Sixteen Drops and

Antarsādhana-Amitāyus are not included in the Hahn Foundation handscrolls. For further comparisons of the *Abhisamayamuktāmālā* and the Hahn Foundation handscrolls, reference should be made to the explanatory remarks on each maṇḍala included in this volume.

The *Vajrāvalī* is a compendium of maṇḍala rituals composed by the Indian Tantric master Abhayākaragupta, who lived in the late eleventh to early twelfth century, and it actually gives detailed descriptions of only twenty-six maṇḍalas. However, according to Professor Mori, variant forms due to the substitution of the central deity and so forth bring the number to forty-two, and if one adds a further three maṇḍalas described in another ritual manual, the *Kriyāsamuccaya*, this results in a total of forty-five maṇḍalas.

Abhayākaragupta also composed two other important manuals, the *Niṣpannayogāvalī* and *Jyotirmañjarī*, as complementary works (*parikara*) to the *Vajrāvalī*. The *Niṣpannayogāvalī* describes characteristics such as the body colour and number of faces and arms for each deity of the twenty-six maṇḍalas explained in the *Vajrāvalī*. Therefore, I have consulted mainly the *Niṣpannayogāvalī* for information on the iconography of each deity.

In addition, lCaṅ skya II, Ṅag dbaṅ blo bzaṅ chos ldan (1642–1714), an eminent monk belonging to the dGe lugs pa order, composed the *rDzogs 'phreṅ daṅ rdor 'phreṅ gñis kyi cho ga phyag len gyi rim pa lag tu blaṅs bde bar dgod pa* (Peking No. 6236), in which he gives detailed explanations of the forty-five maṇḍalas of the *Vajrāvalī*.

The examples of pictorial representations of the *Vajrāvalī* preserved in collections around the world today all depict these forty-five maṇḍalas, and they include sets of thangkas with each thangka depicting one to four maṇḍalas. The oldest extant examples were produced at the start of the fifteenth century at Ṅor monastery, but regrettably this monastery was destroyed during the period between the Tibetan uprising in 1959 and the Cultural Revolution, and the full set no longer exists.

The Hahn Foundation handscrolls, on the other hand, were executed in modern times, but they are not a thangka set or loose-leaf *tsakali*s, and they are complete and depict all the maṇḍalas. In the lower left corner of each maṇḍala the title is written in Tibetan characters (*dbu can* script), and this provides us with firsthand information about the maṇḍalas.

According to the inscriptions, the *Vajrāvalī* depicts forty-five maṇḍalas, starting with the nineteen-deity maṇḍala of Guhyasamāja-Mañjuvajra (V-1) and ending with the maṇḍala of Uṣṇīṣavijayā (V-45). The maṇḍalas are arranged in accordance with the fourfold classification of the tantras, from the Highest Yoga tantras to the Kriyā tantras. The maṇḍalas are arranged in two registers, with only the large-scale Dharmadhātuvāgīśvara-maṇḍala (V-39) occupying both registers.

The *Mitra brgya rtsa*, on the other hand, depicts sixty-five maṇḍalas, starting with the thirteen-deity maṇḍala of Sarasvatī (M-1) and ending with the nine-deity maṇḍala of four-armed Mahākāla (M-65). The maṇḍalas are arranged from the Kriyā tantras to the Highest Yoga tantras, which is the opposite to the order in which they are arranged in the *Vajrāvalī*. The inscriptions give not only the titles but also the number of deities. This is useful for identifying the sixty-five maṇḍalas, which include different maṇḍalas with the same main deity. Moreover, the arrangement of the maṇḍalas coincides not with the *Abhisamayamuktāmālā* but with the Fazangsi lithograph.

Patterns Inside the Square Pavilion

Roṅ tha's Iconometry, mentioned above, classifies the patterns inside the square pavilion (Skt. *kūṭāgāra*) of the maṇḍala into forty-nine categories. A comparison of *Roṅ tha's Iconometry* and the Hahn Foundation handscrolls makes it clear that the patterns inside the square pavilion of the Tibetan maṇḍala consist of three basic patterns, namely, lotus, wheel and nine-panel grid (Skt. *navakoṣṭha*), and combinations thereof.

In the lotus pattern the main deity is depicted on the pericarp of a lotus and the attendants are arranged on the surrounding lotus petals. The number of lotus petals is in many cases eight. But a four-petalled lotus occurs in some cases in Tibet. In Japan, the same pattern of an eight-petalled lotus is seen in the centre of the Garbhadhātu-maṇḍala, while the thirty-five-deity Śākyamuni-maṇḍala (M-6) has a triple eight-petalled pattern. It is interesting that the same pattern occurs in the maṇḍala of Buddhalocanā in Japan.

In the wheel pattern the main deity is depicted on the hub and the attendants are arranged on the spokes. In Tibet, there are patterns of four-, six-, eight- and twelve-spoked wheels. In Japan, on the other hand, this wheel pattern is not often found. The late Professor Shinten Sakai of Kōyasan University pointed out that the maṇḍala in the shape of an eight-spoked wheel originated in the *Prajñāpāramitānaya-sūtra.*

In Japan the wheel (*cakra*) is depicted as the *dharma-cakra* and the attendants are arranged between the spokes. In the Hahn Foundation handscrolls, on the other hand, the wheel is depicted in the shape of the *cakra* as a weapon and the attendants are arranged on the spokes. Maṇḍalas in the shape of the *cakra* as a weapon are frequently encountered not only in Tibet but also in Dunhuang paintings. Therefore, maṇḍalas in the shape of the *cakra* as a weapon also originated in India.

The last pattern, the nine-panel grid, consists of a circle or a square that is divided into a grid of nine sections in which the deities are arranged. In Tibet, this pattern is common in maṇḍalas belonging to the Vajraśekhara cycle, starting with the Vajradhātu-maṇḍala and the Guhyasamāja-maṇḍala.

In maṇḍalas of a complex structure we can see combinations of the above three basic patterns. For example, in the Cakrasaṃvara-maṇḍala (V-19) a triple eight-spoked wheel is arranged around an eight-petalled lotus. The Sarvārthasiddhi-maṇḍala (M-32), a variation of the Vajradhātu-maṇḍala, has a four-petalled lotus in the centre of the nine-panel grid. In addition, maṇḍalas of composite type like the Pañcaḍāka-maṇḍala (V-9) and Ṣaṭcakravartin-maṇḍala (V-26) also can be classified under this category.

In Tibet, there are several maṇḍalas which have unique patterns, such as the crossed vajra (Skt. *viśvavajra*) in the Yamāntaka cycle and a hexagram (Star of David) in the maṇḍala of a Nāropa-style *ḍākinī*. But these are exceptional cases.

The Kāyavākcittapariniṣpanna-Kālacakra-maṇḍala (V-36) is the largest among the many maṇḍalas in Tibet. The iconometry and design of the square pavilion differ considerably from those of other maṇḍalas. But the Hahn Foundation handscrolls depict all the maṇḍalas uniformly, except for the Dharmadhātuvāgīśvara-maṇḍala (V-39).

Tibetan maṇḍalas have an outer protective circle which is not represented in Japanese maṇḍalas, and therefore at first sight they look different from Japanese maṇḍalas. But as regards the pattern inside the square pavilion, Tibetan and Japanese maṇḍalas have much in common. It is particularly interesting that the three basic patterns in Tibetan maṇḍalas, namely, lotus, wheel and nine-panel grid, are the characteristics of the Japanese Garbhadhātu, *Prajñāpāramitānaya-sūtra*, and Vajradhātu maṇḍalas respectively.

Colour Scheme of the Courtyard

Next, let us survey the colour scheme of the courtyard of the maṇḍala. Reference should be made to the diagrams on pp. 14-15.

The centre and four cardinal directions of the courtyard of the Tibetan maṇḍala are painted in accordance with the body colour of the five Buddhas who reside in the centre and four directions of the maṇḍala. Usually the body colours of the five Buddhas are as follows: Vairocana (white), Akṣobhya (blue), Ratnasambhava (yellow), Amitābha (red) and Amoghasiddhi (green). But several tantras explain them differently.

In maṇḍalas of the Yoga tantras, starting with the Vajradhātu-maṇḍala centred on Vairocana, the colour scheme of the courtyard is as follows: centre (white) = Vairocana; east (blue) = Akṣobhya; south (yellow) = Ratnasambhava; west (red) = Amitābha; and north (green) = Amoghasiddhi (cf. Diagram A). In the Hahn Foundation handscrolls, this colour scheme occurs nine times in the Kriyā tantras, nine times in the Yoga tantras, and three times in the Highest Yoga tantras. This means that this colour scheme was also applied to the Kriyā tantras, which represent the early stage of Indian Esoteric Buddhism.

If Vairocana, the main deity of the Yoga tantras, is replaced by Amitābha, the colours of the centre and west are also transposed (cf. Diagram B). This is a characteristic of maṇḍalas of the Lotus family centred on Amitābha, and in the Hahn Foundation handscrolls the maṇḍala of Mahākaruṇika (M-8) and the thirteen-deity maṇḍala of Aparimitāyus (M-24) have this colour scheme.

The Hahn Foundation Handscrolls

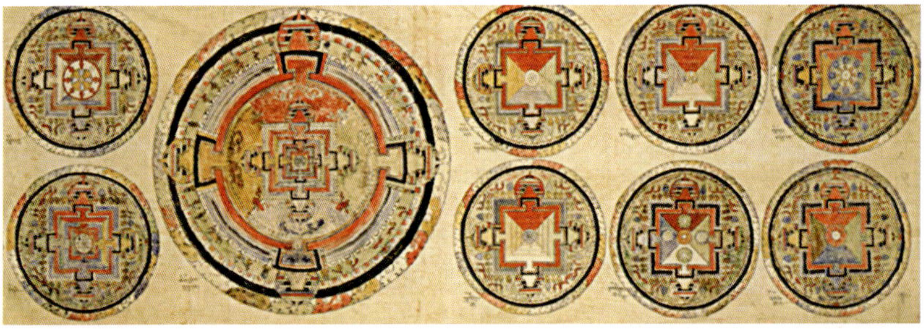

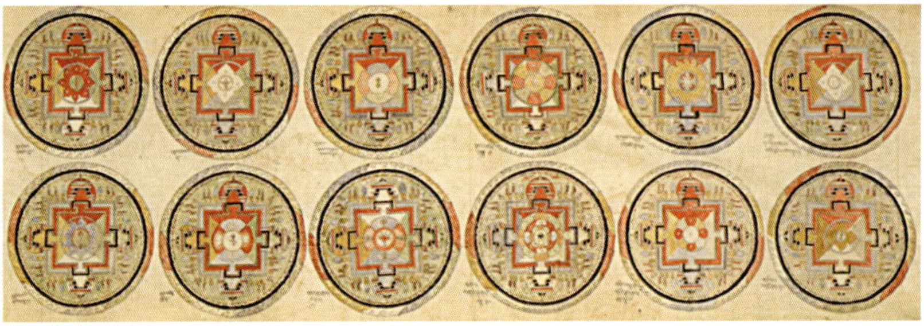

On the other hand, maṇḍalas of the Highest Yoga tantras, starting with the *Guhyasamāja-tantra*, have Akṣobhya as their main deity. The colour scheme of the courtyard is as follows: centre (blue) = Akṣobhya; east (white) = Vairocana; south (yellow) = Ratnasambhava; west (red) = Amitābha; and north (green) = Amoghasiddhi (cf. Diagram E). This colour scheme is the most common, and in the Hahn Foundation handscrolls seventy-one maṇḍalas adopt this colour scheme. The breakdown of these seventy-one maṇḍalas is as follows: twelve in the Kriyā tantras, two in the Caryā tantras, ten in the Yoga tantras, and forty-seven in the Highest Yoga tantras. This means that this colour scheme was applied not only to the Highest Yoga tantras but also to the three lower groups of tantras, which represent the early and middle phases of Esoteric Buddhism.

Moreover, in the Hahn Foundation handscrolls a colour scheme in which Akṣobhya, the main deity of the Highest Yoga tantras, is replaced by Amitābha occurs twice (cf. Diagram F). In both cases, namely, the maṇḍalas of Kurukullā (V-12) and Hayagrīva-Padmanarteśvara (M-63), the main deity belongs to the Lotus family.

In addition, a colour scheme in which Akṣobhya, the main deity of the Highest Yoga tantras, is replaced by Ratnasambhava occurs in five cases (cf. Diagram G). Among these, Vajratārā (V-13), Vasudhārā (V-43) and Yellow Jambhala (M-5) belong to the Jewel family presided over by Ratnasambhava. The colour scheme of the Pañcarakṣā-maṇḍala (V-42) corresponds to the body colour of the five protectresses (Skt. *pañcarakṣā*) arranged in the centre and four cardinal directions. The colour scheme of the thirty-five-deity Śākyamuni-maṇḍala (M-6), on the other hand, seems to follow the colours of the four continents (Skt. *caturdvīpa*) of Abhidharma cosmology.

Furthermore, the Kāyavākcittapariniṣpanna-Kālacakra-maṇḍala (V-36), which represents the final stage of Indian Esoteric Buddhism, adopts a unique colour scheme: center (blue) = Akṣobhya; east (black) = Amoghasiddhi; south (red) = Ratnasambhava; west (yellow) = Vairocana; and north (white) = Amitābha (cf. Diagram D).

In the Hahn Foundation handscrolls, the Vairocana-Mañjuvajra-maṇḍala (V-3), four variations of the nine-deity maṇḍala of Hevajra (V-5~8), and the maṇḍalas of Buddhakapāla (V-32), Jñānaḍākinī (V-35), Navoṣṇīṣa (V-38) and Paramādya-Vajrasattva (M-34), nine maṇḍalas in total, have unique colour schemes which do not belong to any of the above-mentioned schemes.

Some irregular colour schemes found in the Hahn Foundation handscrolls would seem to be due to painting errors. But after further investigations, I discovered that some of them coincide with the textual source of the maṇḍala or with ritual manuals such as the *Niṣpannayogāvalī*. This suggests that these handscrolls were compiled by a Tantric master well-versed in Buddhist iconography.

Image Database of Maṇḍalas Using Computer Graphics

Despite the sketchy quality of the drawings of the maṇḍalas and their pale colours and small size, the Hahn Foundation handscrolls provide us with valuable information for the study of maṇḍalas. Therefore, I decided to create an image database of maṇḍalas using computer graphics by extracting the above-mentioned iconographical information, such as the patterns and colour schemes of the square pavilion.

Tibetan and Nepalese maṇḍalas in particular are characterized by a geometrical layout that is completely symmetrical, both horizontally and vertically, and by the repetition of certain patterns. In maṇḍala collections, moreover, in which the images need to be recorded accurately, it is desirable not only for the differences between individual maṇḍalas to be depicted accurately, but also for elements common to all the maṇḍalas to be shown uniformly without any variation. In this respect, an image database of maṇḍalas could be described as an ideal subject for computer graphics.

Computer graphics software can be broadly divided into drawing software and painting software. Drawing software uses a system of coordinates to record data, and it therefore has the advantage of being able to output smooth circles, curves, etc., even at extremely high resolutions. But the production of high-resolution computer graphics with drawing software requires a high level of CPU performance.

Furthermore, complete compatibility of data cannot be guaranteed between different types of drawing software. Especially in the case of maṇḍalas, with their complex gradation and texture, data conversion can result in an enormous increase in data, with the individual gradation levels and textured sections being resolved into complex polygons.

Painting software, on the other hand, uses a number of common formats such as GIF, BMP and TIFF, depending on the number of colours and the resolution, and data compatibility is ensured. Moreover, since gradation and texture are output in the form of pixels, painting software places no extra burden on CPU usage.

In light of these differences between drawing software and painting software, I accordingly adopted a method whereby I used drawing software to produce only the contours of the maṇḍalas, with their complex layout, which were then converted into image data of a suitable pixel count in accordance with the printout size, while painting software was used to create the colours requiring gradation and texture.

Even if the performance of computers and printers should improve in the future, thereby making it possible to produce data of still greater pixel counts, with this method it will be possible to utilize the data produced with drawing software as it is or with only minor refinements. When data of 18,000,000 pixels is printed with the largest commercially available printer on paper 1.1 m square, no jaggedness arising from the fact that the data is pixel data is noticeable unless one looks very carefully at the printout.

When creating the CG maṇḍalas, I adopted the method of creating an outer enclosure shared by all the maṇḍalas apart from the Dharmadhātuvāgīśvara-maṇḍala (V-39) and substituting different images of the *toraṇa* and the inside of the pavilion depending on the maṇḍala. For the *Vajrāvalī* and *Mitra brgya rtsa* I used different textures and designs for the texture of the outer perimeter and the design of the banners and parasols placed on top of the pavilion. Further, the *Vajrāvalī* gives detailed instructions regarding the design of the different parts of the maṇḍala, but the *Abhisamayamuktāmālā* makes almost no mention of the pavilion. Therefore, a considerable degree of conjectural reconstruction was needed in the case of details of the pavilion not described in the original texts.

Meanwhile, when the prescriptions found in the Hahn Foundation handscrolls and the *Vajrāvalī* differed, priority was given to the form of expression found in the Hahn Foundation handscrolls except in cases of obvious errors. But when the number of deities mentioned in the text or inscription was greater than the number depicted in the maṇḍala, extra places were added in suitable positions.

In the case of smaller works such as maṇḍala collections, the four quarters of the courtyard of the pavilion are often painted in a single colour without any texture or gradation. In the present instance, I created several different textures with reference to the Ṅor maṇḍalas which I then used as appropriate. This was done in order to add variation to maṇḍalas of the same pattern. Further, in the case of maṇḍalas in which symbols are depicted in the courtyard, a light colour was used for the texture so as to make it easier to distinguish the symbols.

Exhibiting CG Maṇḍalas

In 2001, I first created some CG maṇḍalas and used them as illustrations for the catalogue of the Hahn Cultural Foundation's exhibition in Japan, "The World of Thangka." However, the number of pixels per maṇḍala was a mere 1,300,000.

In 2003 I created a new image database of the maṇḍalas in the *Mitra brgya rtsa* using computer graphics and exhibited it at the annual exhibition held at the Meditation Museum in Toga Village, Toyama Prefecture, where I am chief curator. On that occasion, the number of pixels reached 5,000,000, about three times more than before. We used dye inks for the printouts, and because of discoloration we had to remove all the maṇḍalas after half a year.

In 2004, several CG maṇḍalas were put on display at the International Mountain Museum in Pokhara, Nepal, and the forty-five maṇḍalas of the *Vajrāvalī* were exhibited on the occasion of "The World of Maṇḍalas" exhibition held at the Ōkura Shūkokan (Tokyo) in 2005 and were well received by visitors.

After making further improvements to the data, such as raising the resolution of complex maṇḍalas to 18,000,000 pixels, I again exhibited them at the Meditation Museum in 2006. This time, we printed them out with pigment inks, and according to the maker the ink should last for ten years. They have, therefore, become a permanent exhibit at the Meditation Museum. The 108 maṇḍalas are exhibited in the following manner: four large-size maṇḍalas, namely, Dharmadhātuvāgīśvara (V-39), Ṣaṭcakravartin (V-26), Pañcaḍāka (V-9) and Kāyavākcittapariniṣpanna-Kālacakra (V-36), have been placed in the centre of the four walls in the north, east, west and south respectively, while the other 104 maṇḍalas have been arranged around these four maṇḍalas (cf. photograph on p. 13).

The Structure of This Book

This book is an English version of my *Maṇḍala Graphics*, which was published in Japanese in April 2007 by Yamakawa Publications (Tokyo).

Each page contains one CG maṇḍala based on the Hahn Foundation handscrolls, and each maṇḍala is accompanied by explanatory remarks. The inscription in Tibetan script (bottom left) is a transcription of the inscription in the original handscroll. Some of these inscriptions are problematic, but they have not been corrected except in cases of obvious errors. However, shortened words (*skuṅ yig*) appearing in the original inscriptions have been written out in full.

The name of the maṇḍala in English appears at the top left. In addition, the number and category of the patterns inside the square pavilion, based on *Roṅ tha's Iconometry,* and the colour scheme of the courtyard, such as "Yoga tantras centred on Vairocana," is given at the top

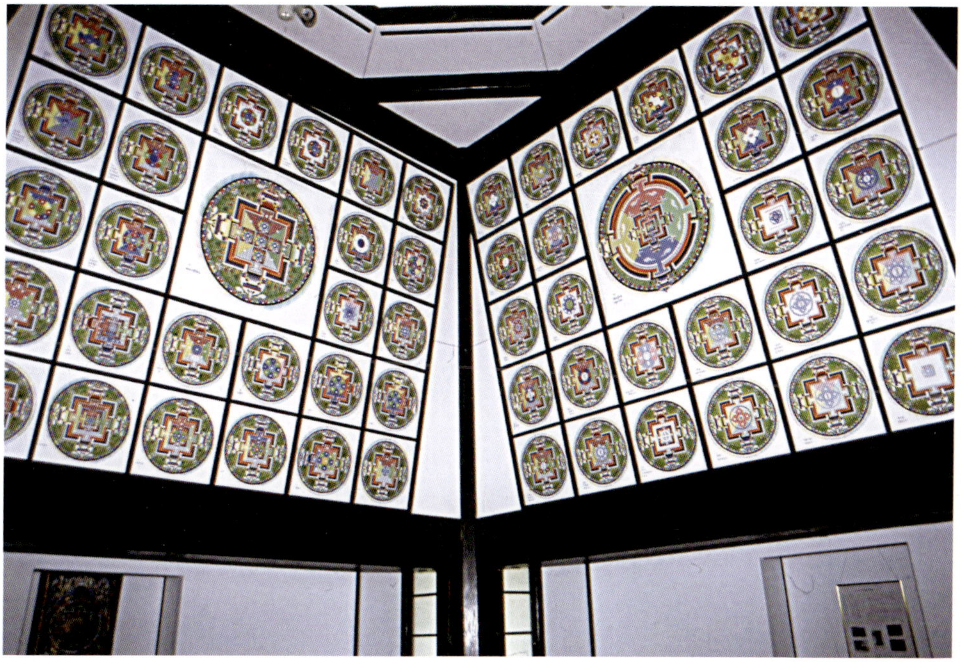

Toga Meditation Museum

right. At the bottom right is the number of the maṇḍala as it appears in the textual sources, namely, the *Abhisamayamuktāmālā* (AMM) and *Vajrāvalī* (VA).

Maṇḍalas are not merely magnificent works of art, but embody the ideas and cosmology of Buddhism. They have also attracted attention as cosmograms that show the world of reality or psychograms that illustrate the structure of the human mind. Commercially, too, maṇḍalas have become popular as cuts and illustrations for books, designs for posters, and materials for jigsaw puzzles and colouring books.

As a result of the Tibetan uprising in 1959 and the Cultural Revolution in the 1960s to 1970s, the basic materials for the study of Tibetan Buddhist iconography, such as maṇḍala sets, became scattered far and wide and are now found in collections around the world. Unfortunately, most of these works remain unidentified.

In such circumstances, the publication of this image database of Mitrayogin's 108 maṇḍalas, representing the final stage of development of the maṇḍala in India, should be of considerable value. I very much hope that the publication of this book will contribute to further understanding of Tibetan Buddhism and its maṇḍalas.

Lastly, I would like to offer my heartful thanks to all those who helped in the preparation of this publication, including Rolf W. Giebel, who supervised the English translation, the Japan Society for the Promotion of Science, which provided financial support for the translation work, and Bidul Dangol, president of Vajra Publications, who undertook to publish this book with great care.

Colour Schemes of the Courtyard (1)

A. Yoga tantras

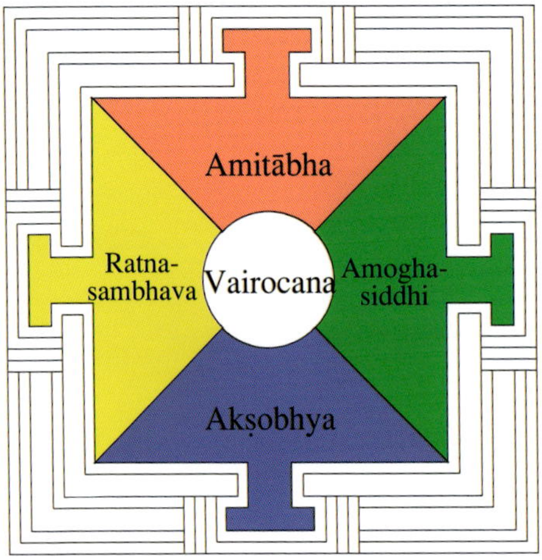

C. Māyājāla-tantra

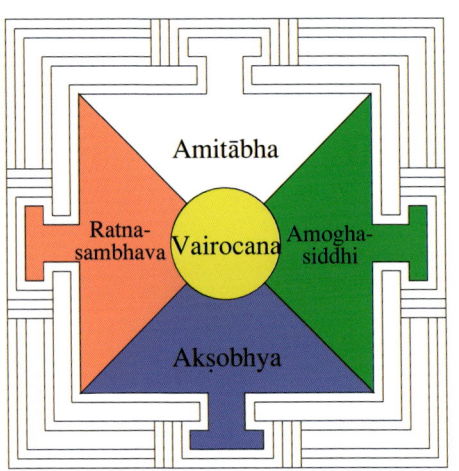

B. Yoga tantras centred on Amitābha

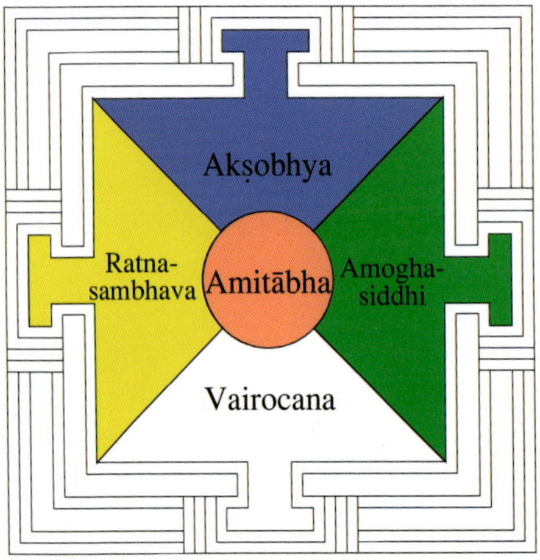

D. Kālacakra-tantra

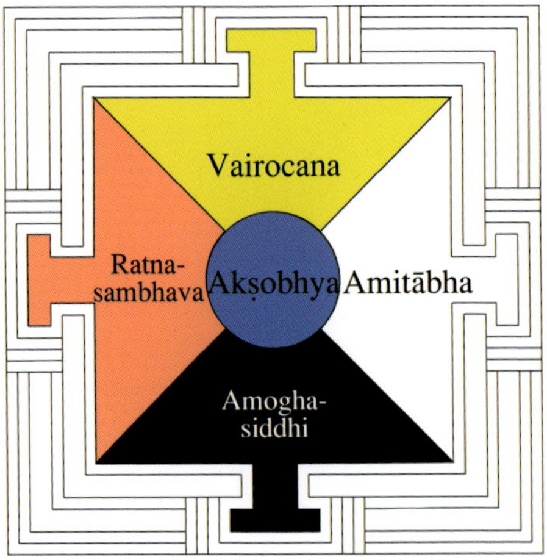

Colour Schemes of the Courtyard (2)

E. Highest Yoga tantras

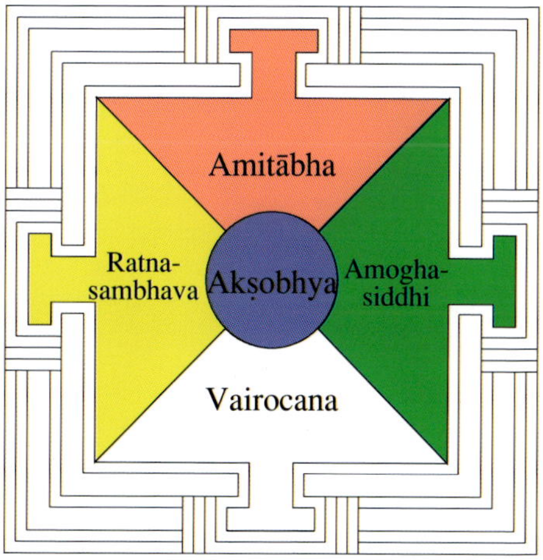

G. Highest Yoga tantras
centred on Ratnasambhava

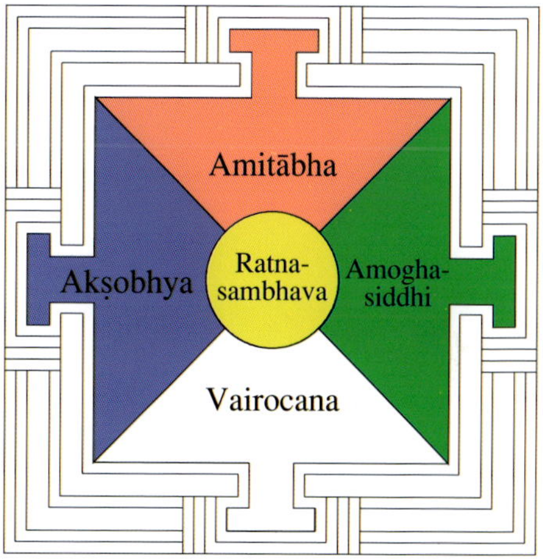

F. Highest Yoga tantras
centred on Amitābha

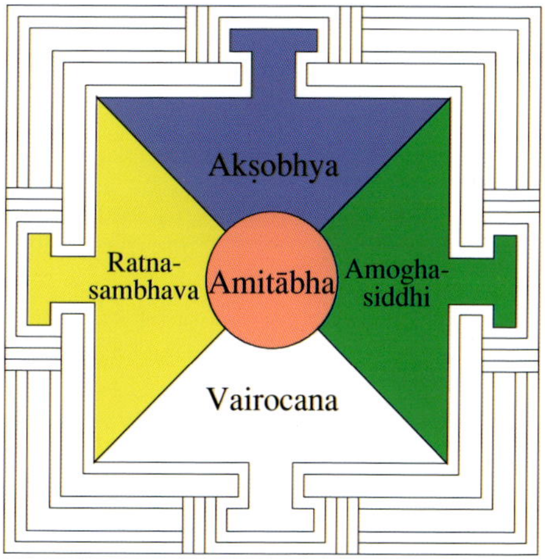

H. Nine-deity Hevajra-maṇḍala

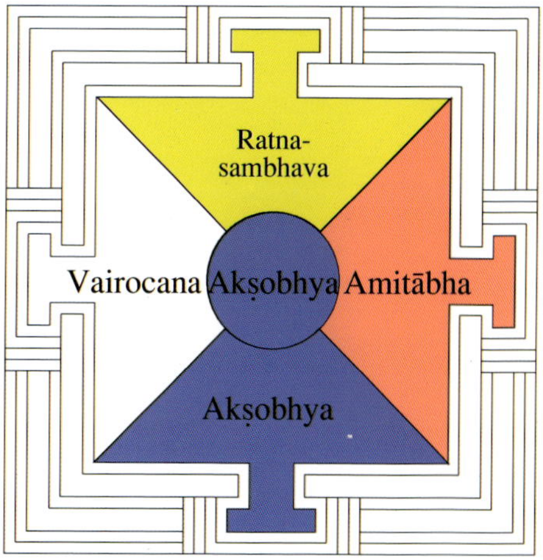

Explanatory Remarks on
the *Vajrāvalī* Set of Maṇḍalas

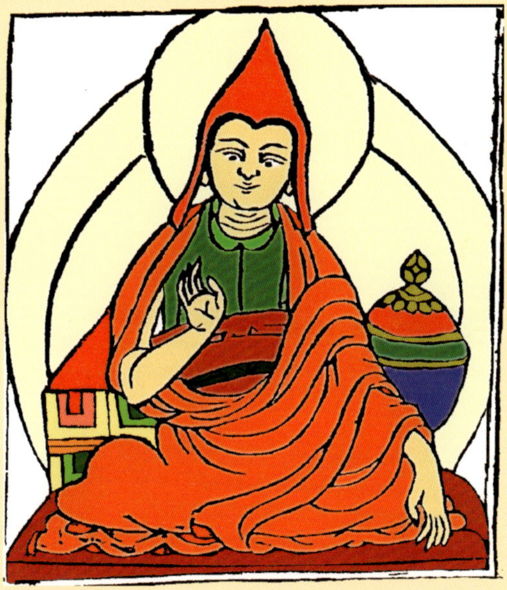

Abhayākaragupta, the author of the *Vajrāvalī*

1. Nineteen-deity Guhyasamāja-Mañjuvajra-maṇḍala

Pattern: 1. Nine-panel grid;
Colour scheme:
Highest Yoga tantras
centred on Akṣobhya

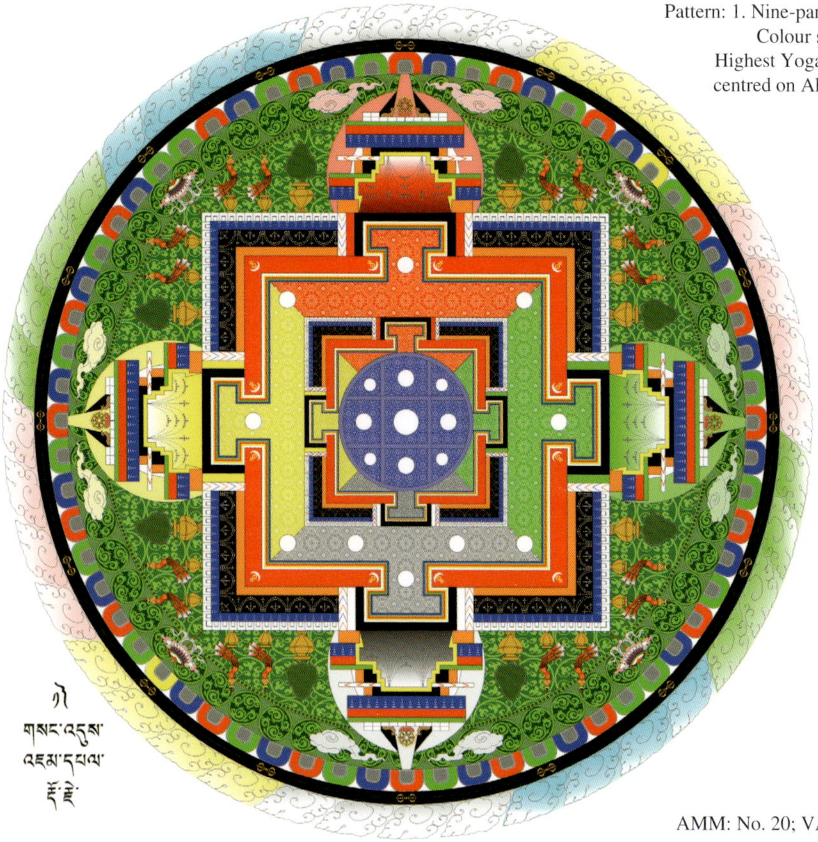

༡༽
གསང་འདུས་
འཇམ་དཔལ་
རྡོ་རྗེ་

AMM: No. 20; VA: No. 1

The *Guhyasamāja-tantra* is a representative scripture of late Tantric Buddhism, and this maṇḍala belongs to the Jñānapāda school among the two major schools of interpretation of the *Guhyasamāja-tantra*. The centre of the maṇḍala takes the form of a nine-panel grid, with Vairocana (east), Ratnaketu (south), Amitābha (west) and Amoghasiddhi (north) in the four cardinal directions around the main deity. In the four intermediate directions of the central circle are Locanā (southeast), Māmakī (southwest), Pāṇḍarā (northwest) and Tārā (northeast). Outside the central square are the six adamantine goddesses Rūpavajrā (southeast), Śabdavajrā (southwest), Gandhavajrā (northwest), Rasavajrā (northeast), Sparśavajrā (north side of east gate) and Dharmadhātuvajrā (south side of west gate), and in the four gates are the four wrathful deities Yamāntaka (east), Prajñāntaka (south), Padmāntaka (west) and Vighnāntaka (north). Thus, this maṇḍala consists of nineteen deities. The colour scheme of the courtyard is that of the Highest Yoga tantras centred on Akṣobhya (Type E), which was also widely adopted in other maṇḍalas belonging to the Highest Yoga tantras. In the Hahn Foundation handscroll, this maṇḍala is depicted as a double pavilion, contrary to the norm, and the seats for the six adamantine goddesses are also missing. These latter have, however, been added with reference to the *Niṣpannayogāvalī*.

2. Thirty-two-deity Guhyasamāja-Akṣobhyavajra-maṇḍala

Pattern: 1. Nine-panel grid;
Colour scheme:
Highest Yoga tantras
centred on Akṣobhya

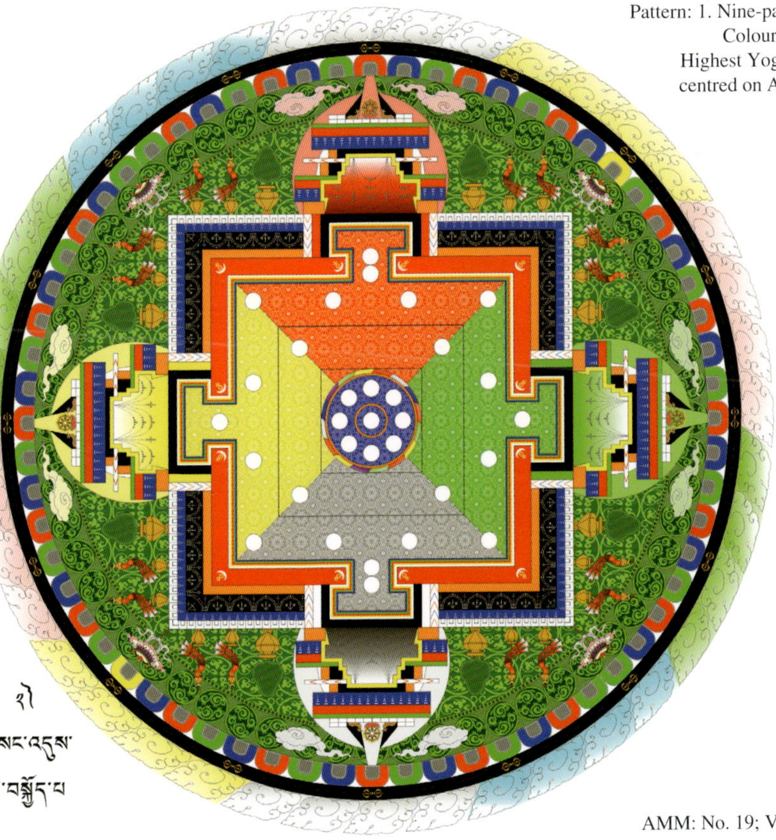

༢།
གསང་འདུས་
མི་བསྐྱོད་པ

AMM: No. 19; VA: No. 2

This maṇḍala belongs to the Ārya school, one of the two major schools of interpretation of the *Guhyasamāja-tantra*. The central circle of the maṇḍala takes the form of a nine-panel grid. In the centre of the circle, the main deity Akṣobhyavajra is depicted together with his consort Sparśavajrā, both three-headed and six-armed. Vairocana (east), Ratnaketu (south), Amitābha (west) and Amoghasiddhi (north) are arranged in the four cardinal directions around the main deity, and in the four intermediate directions of the central circle are Locanā (southeast), Māmakī (southwest), Pāṇḍarā (northwest) and Tārā (northeast). Rūpavajrā (southeast), Śabdavajrā (southwest), Gandhavajrā (northwest) and Rasavajrā (northeast) occupy the four corners of the inner square. In the outer square are the eight great bodhisattvas Maitreya, Kṣitigarbha (east), Vajrapāṇi, Ākāśagarbha (south), Lokeśvara, Mañjuśrī (west), Sarvanīvaraṇaviṣkambhin and Samantabhadra (north) and also the ten wrathful deities Yamāntaka (east gate), Prajñāntaka (south gate), Padmāntaka (west gate), Vighnāntaka (north gate), Acala (southeast corner), Ṭakkirāja (southwest corner), Nīladaṇḍa (northwest corner), Mahābala (northeast corner), Uṣṇīṣacakravartin (top) and Sumbharāja (bottom). Thus, this maṇḍala consists of thirty-two deities. The iconometry and the design of the gates of the maṇḍala in the Hahn Foundation handscroll differ from the norms of the Ārya school, but the original has been followed here. The colour scheme of the courtyard is that of the Highest Yoga tantras centred on Akṣobhya (Type E).

3. Forty-three-deity Vairocana-Mañjuvajra-maṇḍala

Pattern: 6. Nine-panel grid;
Colour scheme: Māyājāla

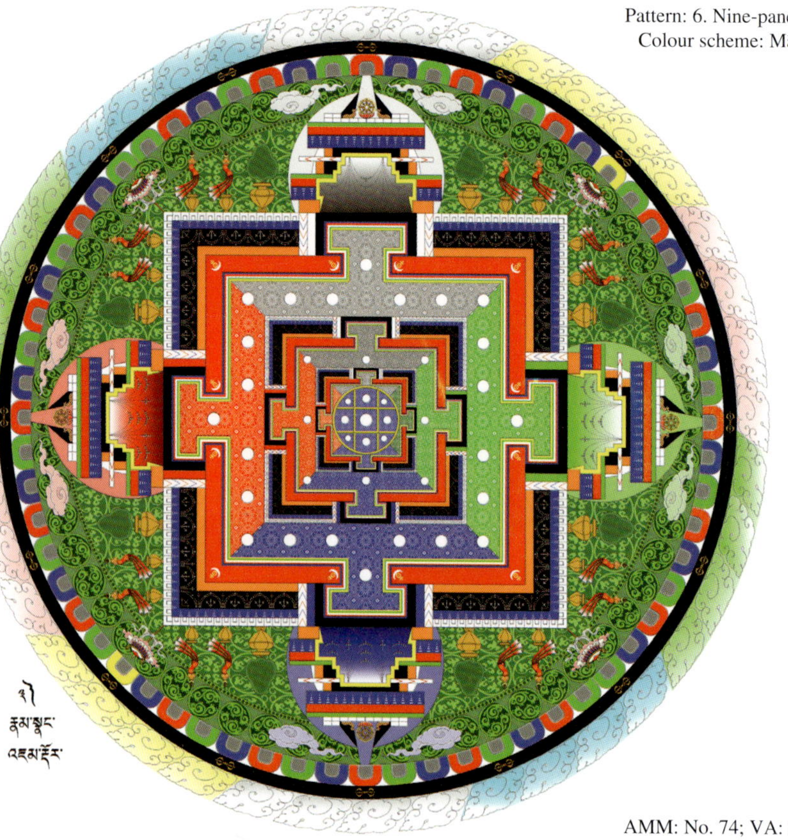

AMM: No. 74; VA: No. 20

This maṇḍala is described in the *Māyājāla-tantra*. Three-headed and six-armed Mañjuvajra is depicted as the main deity in the centre of a nine-panel grid inside a triple pavilion. Akṣobhya (east), Ratnasambhava (south), Amitābha (west) and Amoghasiddhi (north) are arranged in the four cardinal directions around the main deity, while the four Buddha-mothers are arranged in the intermediate directions of the nine-panel grid. The reason that the main deity is called "Vairocana-Mañjuvajra" is that, whereas in the *Guhyasamāja-tantra* Mañjuvajra corresponds to Akṣobhya, in this maṇḍala he corresponds to Vairocana. The second square depicts the four *pāramitā* goddesses starting with Sattvavajrī in the four cardinal directions and four female deities—Cundā (northeast), Ratnolkā (southeast), Bhṛkuṭī (southwest) and Vajraśṛṅkhalā (northwest)—in the four intermediate directions. The third square consists of the sixteen bodhisattvas of the Auspicious Aeon (Bhadrakalpa), although they differ somewhat from those in the Vajradhātu-maṇḍala, and ten wrathful deities (almost identical with those in the Guhyasamāja-Akṣobhyavajra-maṇḍala). The *Abhisamayamuktāmālā* gives the number of deities as forty-two, but this has been corrected to forty-three with reference to the *Patraratnamālā*. Although many other examples of this maṇḍala adopt the courtyard colour scheme of the Yoga tantras, centred on Vairocana (Type A), the Hahn Foundation handscroll adopts an unusual colour scheme (Type C) based on the *Māyājāla-tantra*.

4. Thirteen-deity Kṛṣṇayamāri-maṇḍala

Pattern: 8. Crossed vajra;
Colour scheme:
Highest Yoga tantras
centred on Akṣobhya

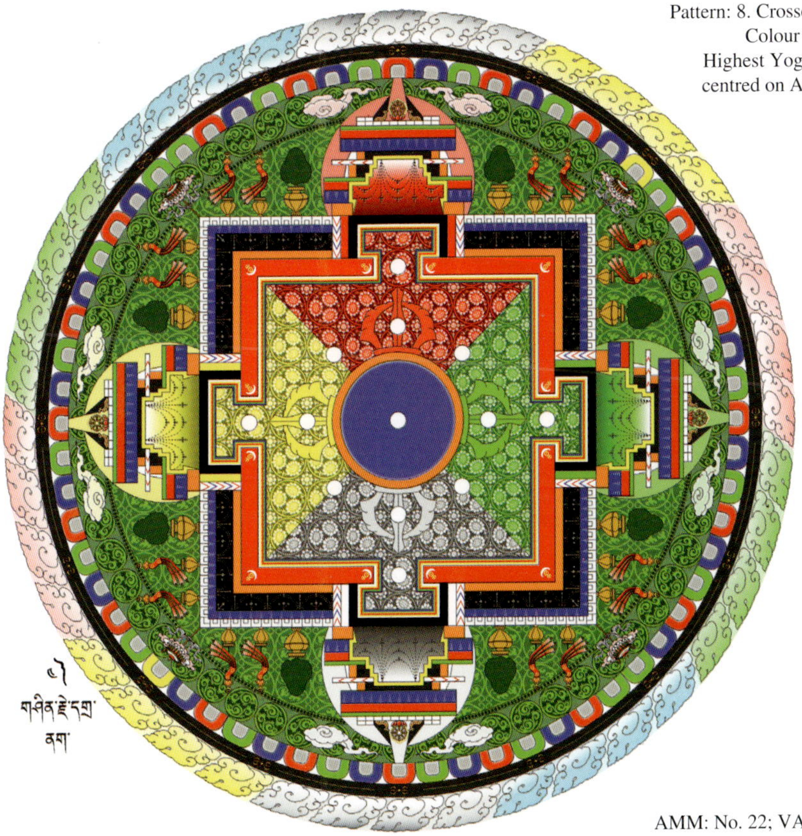

༤།
གཤིན་རྗེ་དགྲ་
ནག་

AMM: No. 22; VA: No. 15

Kṛṣṇayamāri means "black enemy of Yama (god of death)" and is thought to be a form of Yamāntaka, the "destroyer of Yama." In Tibet, three styles of Yamāntaka (*gŚin rje dmar nag 'jigs gsum*), namely, Raktayamāri, Kṛṣṇayamāri and Vajrabhairava, are worshipped as the main deity in rites of subjugation (*abhicāraka*) to defeat the enemies of Buddhism. This maṇḍala takes the form of a wheel with four spokes in the shape of a crossed vajra. In the centre the main deity Kṛṣṇayamāri, three-headed, six-armed and blue in colour, is depicted together with his consort Vajravetālī. Mohayamāri (east), Matsaryayamāri (south), Rāgayamāri (west) and Īrṣyāyamāri (north) are arranged on the spokes in the four cardinal directions. Between the spokes are the four wrathful goddesses Carcikā (southeast), Vārāhī (southwest), Sarasvatī (northwest) and Gaurī (northeast). In the four gates are four gatekeepers, starting with Mudgarayamāri. Although the version in the Hahn Foundation handscroll does not depict a crossed vajra, the characteristic feature of this maṇḍala, it has been supplemented with reference to other examples of this maṇḍala. The colour scheme of the courtyard is that of the Highest Yoga tantras centred on Akṣobhya (Type E).

5. Nine-deity Garbha-Hevajra-maṇḍala

Pattern: 15. Eight-petalled lotus;
Colour scheme: Hevajra

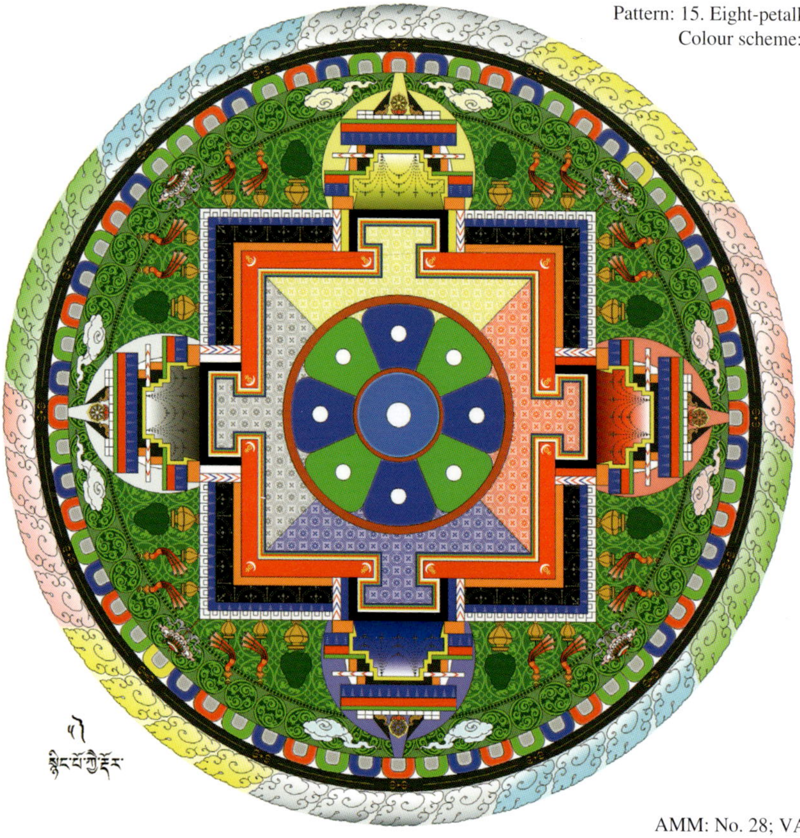

སྙིང་པོ་ཀྱེ་རྡོར་

AMM: No. 28; VA: No. 8a

The *Hevajra-tantra*, along with the *Saṃvara-tantra*, is a representative Mother tantra of the Highest Yoga tantras. The Hevajra-maṇḍala has various styles, among which this maṇḍala is the most popular. It takes the form of an eight-petalled lotus, on the pericarp of which Hevajra, eight-headed, sixteen-armed and four-legged, is depicted embraced by his one-headed and two-armed consort Nairātmyā. On the eight lotus petals are the eight goddesses Gaurī (east), Caurī (south), Vetālī (west), Ghasmarī (north), Pukkasī (northeast), Śabarī (southeast), Caṇḍālī (southwest) and Ḍombī (northwest). In other examples of this maṇḍala, the colour scheme of the courtyard is that of the Highest Yoga tantras centred on Akṣobhya (Type E) since Hevajra belongs to the Vajra family headed by Akṣobhya. The Hahn Foundation handscroll, on the other hand, adopts an unusual colour scheme consisting of blue (east), white (south), yellow (west) and red (north) (Type H). This might be based on the description in the *Niṣpannayogāvalī*, according to which the four goddesses in the cardinal directions, starting with Gaurī, correspond to Akṣobhya, Vairocana, Ratnasambhava and Amitābha respectively. Therefore, this colour scheme may not be an error. This suggests that this handscroll was compiled by a Tantric master well-versed in Buddhist iconography.

6. Nine-deity Citta-Hevajra-maṇḍala

Pattern: 15. Eight-petalled lotus;
Colour scheme: Hevajra

༦
ཐུགས་ཀྱི་
ཀྱཻ་རྡོར་

AMM: No. 29; VA: No. 8b

The *Hevajra-tantra*, along with the *Saṃvara-tantra*, is a representative Mother tantra of the Highest Yoga tantras. The Hevajra-maṇḍala has various styles, among which this maṇḍala is called "Citta-Hevajra," or "Mind-Hevajra," because it is assigned to the mind among the three mysteries of body, speech and mind. It is a variant form of the nine-deity Garbha-Hevajra-maṇḍala (V-5) in which eight-headed, sixteen-armed and four-legged Hevajra has been replaced as the main deity by a form of Hevajra with three heads—blue (front), white (right) and red (left)—and six arms. He is embracing his consort Vajraśṛṅkhalā with two of his arms and holding a vajra and a *kartṛ* in his two other right hands and a trident and a bell in his two other left hands. Accordingly, the pattern and the colour scheme of the courtyard ought to be the same as V-5 (Type H). However, the Hahn Foundation handscroll adopts an unusual colour scheme consisting of blue (east), yellow (south), white (west) and red (north). But this has been changed so as to agree with V-5 since the colour scheme of the Hahn Foundation handscroll is probably an error.

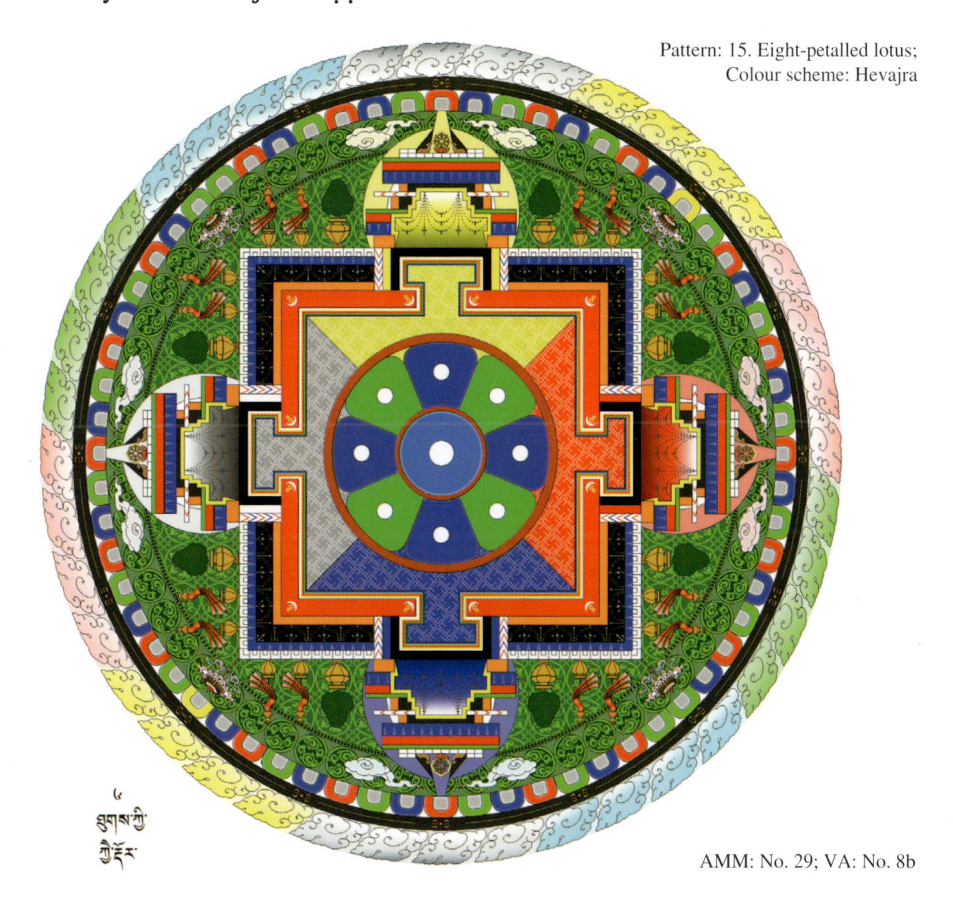

7. Nine-deity Vāk-Hevajra-maṇḍala

Pattern: 15. Eight-petalled lotus;
Colour scheme: Hevajra

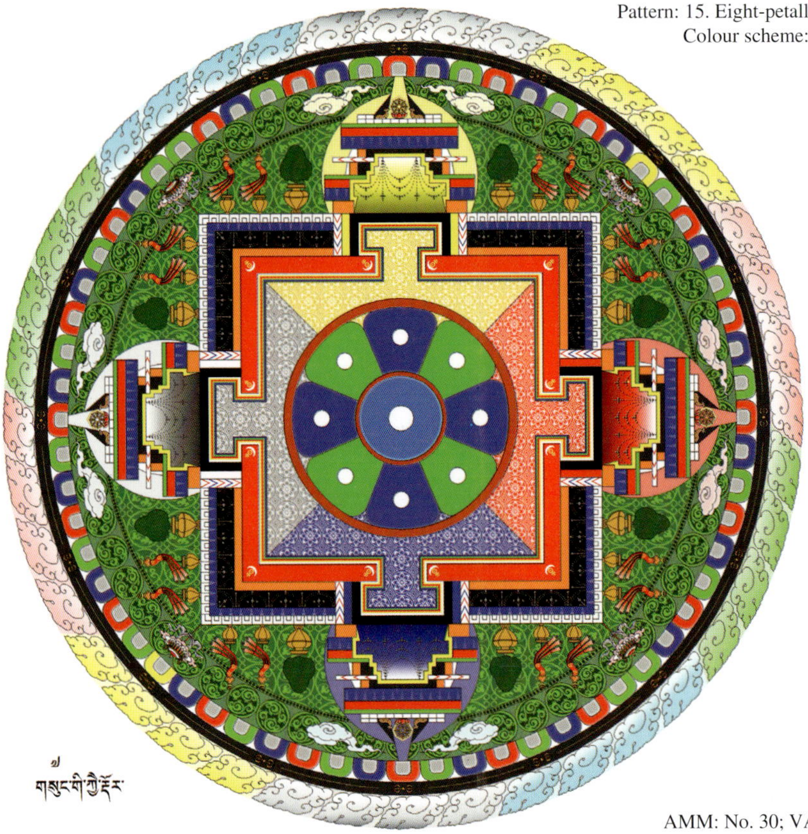

༧
གསུང་གི་ཀྱཻ་རྡོར་

AMM: No. 30; VA: No. 8c

The Hevajra-maṇḍala has various styles, among which this maṇḍala is called "Vāk-Hevajra," or "Speech-Hevajra," because it is assigned to speech among the three mysteries of body, speech and mind. It is a variant form of the nine-deity Garbha-Hevajra-maṇḍala (V-5) in which eight-headed, sixteen-armed and four-legged Hevajra has been replaced as the main deity by a one-headed and four-armed form of Hevajra who is embracing his consort Vajraśṛṅkhalā with his two main arms and holding a vajra and a *kapāla* (skull cup) in his other two right hands and also in his other two left hands. Accordingly, the pattern is a form of the eight-petalled lotus, and the colour scheme of the courtyard is the same as V-5 (Type H).

8. Nine-deity Kāya-Hevajra-maṇḍala

Pattern: 15. Eight-petalled lotus;
Colour scheme: Hevajra

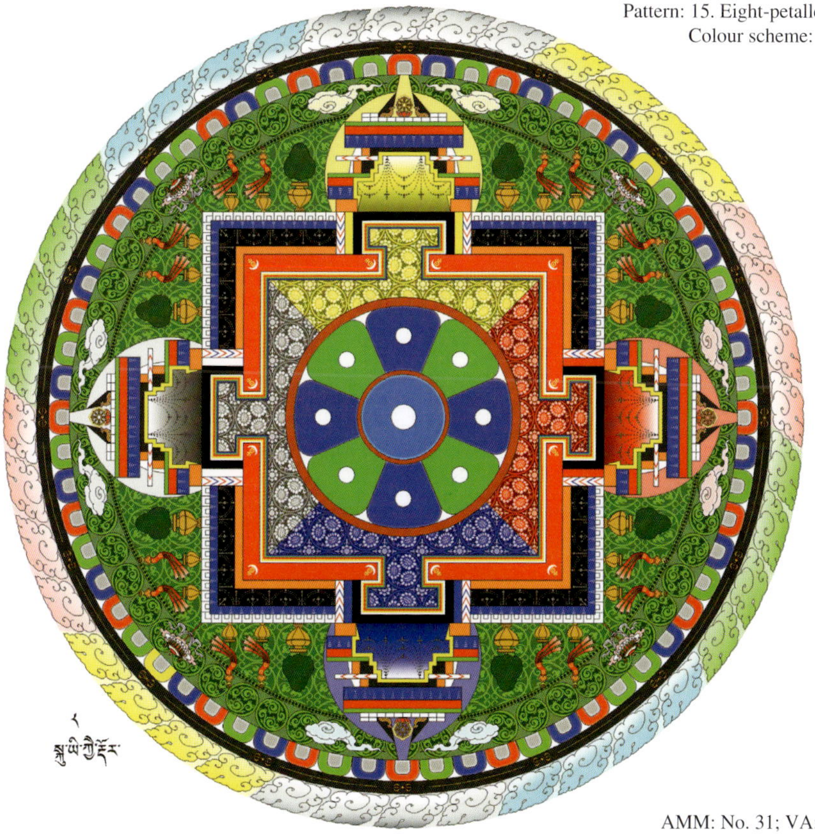

༨
སྐུ་ཡི་ཀྱཻ་རྡོར་

AMM: No. 31; VA: No. 8d

The Hevajra-maṇḍala has various styles, among which this maṇḍala is called "Kāya-Hevajra," or "Body-Hevajra," because it is assigned to the body among the three mysteries of body, speech and mind. It is a variant form of the nine-deity Garbha-Hevajra-maṇḍala (V-5) in which eight-headed, sixteen-armed and four-legged Hevajra has been replaced as the main deity by a one-headed and two-armed form of Hevajra who is embracing his consort Nairātmyā and holding a vajra and a *kapāla* in his right and left hands respectively. Accordingly, the pattern is a form of the eight-petalled lotus, and the colour scheme of the courtyard is the same as V-5 (Type H).

9. Pañcaḍāka-maṇḍala

Pattern: Composite type;
Colour scheme:
Highest Yoga tantras
centred on Akṣobhya

༩་
མཁའ་འགྲོ་སྡེ་ལྔ་

AMM: Nos. 46-50; VA: No. 24

The Pañcaḍāka-maṇḍala is a development of the Hevajra-maṇḍala and is described in the *Vajrapañjara-tantra*, an explanatory tantra of the Hevajra cycle. Pañcaḍāka means "five *ḍāka*s (male form of *ḍākinī*)," and this maṇḍala consists of five small maṇḍalas, each depicting in the centre as the main deity one of the five *ḍāka*s—Vajraḍāka (centre), Buddhaḍāka (east), Ratnaḍāka (south), Padmaḍāka (west) and Viśvaḍāka (north)—along with their consorts. The *Abhisamayamuktāmālā* treats these maṇḍalas as five independent maṇḍalas (Nos. 46-50). The five *ḍāka*s are surrounded by eight *ḍākinī*s, and Vajraḍāka in the centre is surrounded by the same eight female deities as appear in the nine-deity Hevajra-maṇḍalas (V-5~8). Therefore, this maṇḍala can be understood as a fivefold expansion of the nine-deity Hevajra-maṇḍala. In addition, eight *ḍākinī*s are arranged in the four cardinal and four intermediate directions of the outer square. Thus, the total number of deities is fifty-three, and if the consorts of the five *ḍāka*s are included, it becomes fifty-eight. The colour scheme of the courtyard is that of the Highest Yoga tantras centred on Akṣobhya (Type E).

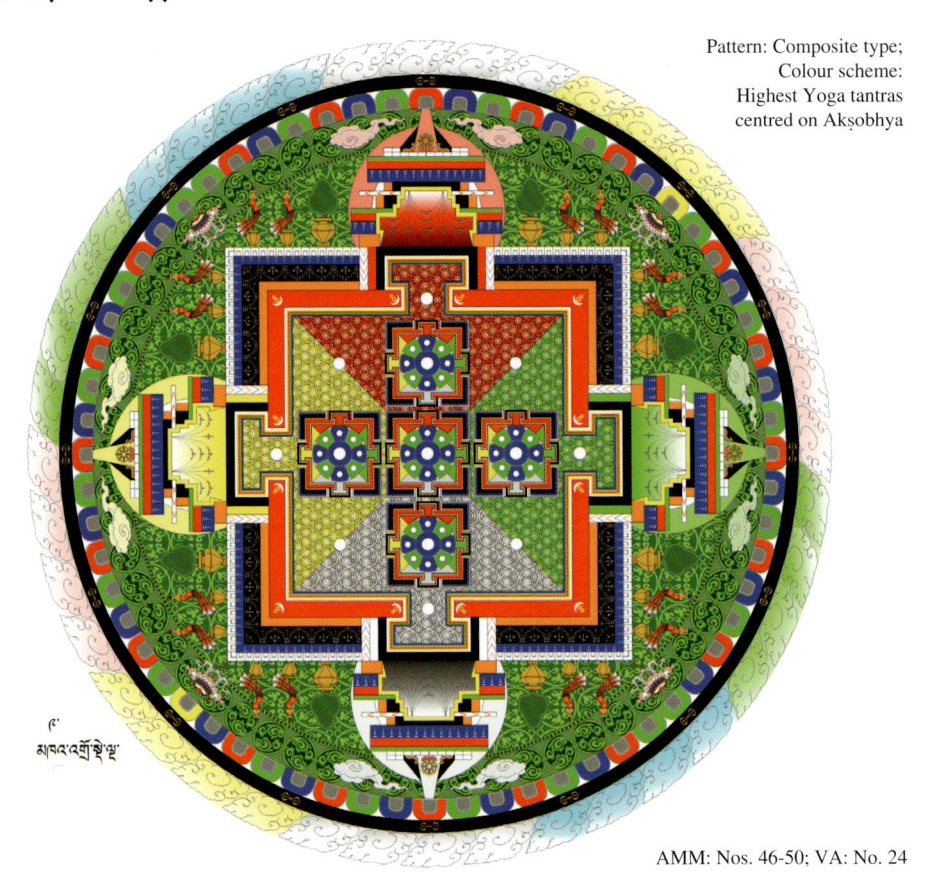

10. Twenty-three-deity Nairātmyā-maṇḍala

Pattern: 19. Eight-petalled lotus;
Colour scheme:
Highest Yoga tantras
centred on Akṣobhya

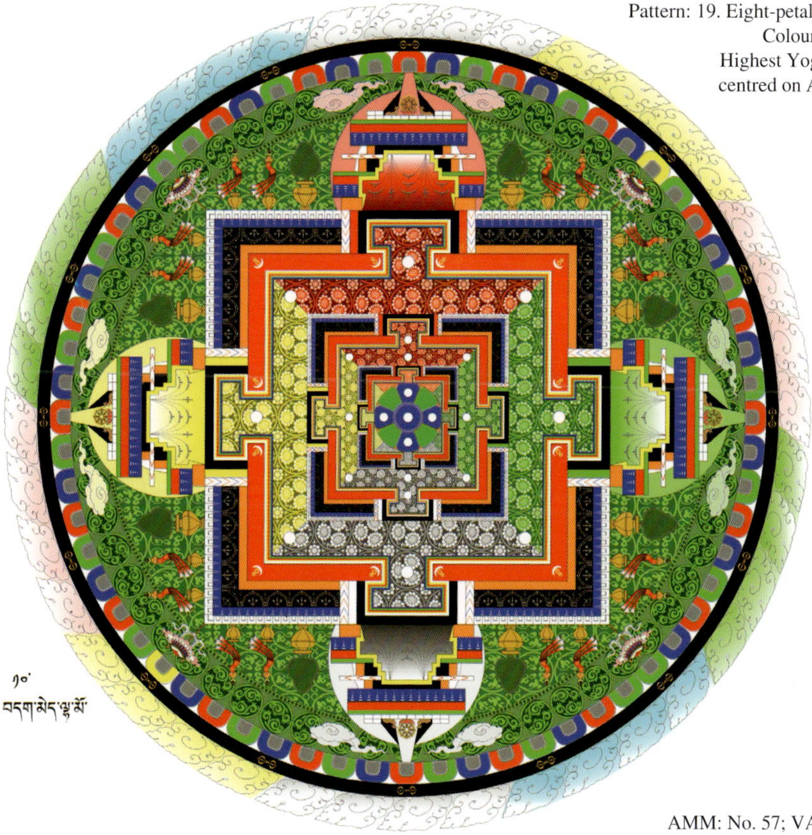

༡༠་
བདག་མེད་ལྷ་མོ་

AMM: No. 57; VA: No. 6a

The maṇḍala of Nairātmyā, a consort of Hevajra, has various styles, among which this maṇḍala is expounded in the *Saṃpuṭa-tantra*, an explanatory tantra of the *Hevajra-tantra* and *Saṃvara-tantra*. This maṇḍala depicts the main deity, Nairātmyā, in the centre of an eight-petalled lotus inside a triple pavilion. Vajrā (east), Gaurī (south), Vārī (west) and Vajraḍākinī (north) are arranged on four lotus petals surrounding the main deity. In the second square are the ten goddesses Gaurī (east), Caurī (south), Vetālī (west), Ghasmarī (north), Pukkasī (northeast), Śabarī (southeast), Caṇḍālī (southwest), Ḍombī (northwest), Khecarī (top) and Bhūcarī (bottom). In the outermost square are four animal-headed female gatekeepers, starting with Hayāsyā (east), and four goddesses of musical instruments, i.e., Vaṃśā (northeast), Vīṇā (southeast), Mukundā (southwest) and Murajā (northwest). In the Hahn Foundation handscroll, this maṇḍala lacks the seats for Khecarī and Bhūcarī, and they have been added with reference to other examples. The colour scheme of the courtyard is that of the Highest Yoga tantras centred on Akṣobhya (Type E).

11. Fifteen-deity Nairātmyā-maṇḍala

Pattern: 19. Eight-petalled lotus;
Colour scheme:
Highest Yoga tantras
centred on Akṣobhya

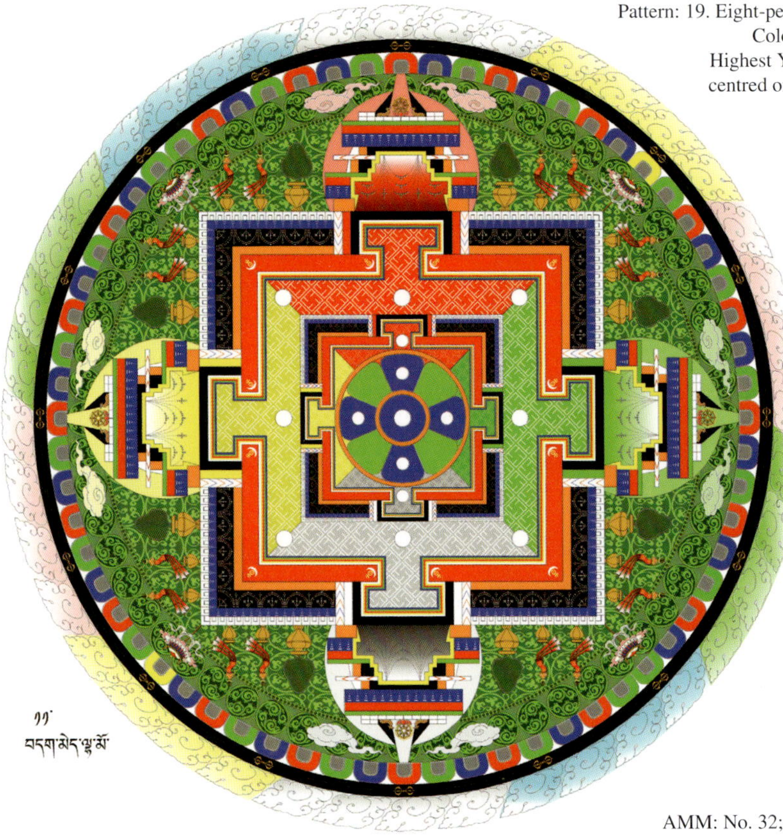

༡༡
བདག་མེད་ལྷ་མོ

AMM: No. 32; VA: No. 6b

The maṇḍala of Nairātmyā, a consort of Hevajra, has various styles, among which this maṇḍala depicts the main deity Nairātmyā in the centre of an eight-petalled lotus inside a double pavilion. Vajrā (east), Gaurī (south), Vārī (west) and Vajraḍākinī (north) are arranged on four lotus petals surrounding the main deity. In the outer square are the ten goddesses Gaurī (east), Caurī (south), Vetālī (west), Ghasmarī (north), Pukkasī (northeast), Śabarī (southeast), Caṇḍālī (southwest), Ḍombī (northwest), Khecarī (top) and Bhūcarī (bottom). This corresponds to the twenty-three-deity Nairātmyā-maṇḍala (V-10) without the outermost square. The *Saṃpuṭa-tantra* (III.iii), thought to be the textual source for this maṇḍala, describes only fifteen deities, and the remaining eight goddesses in the outermost square were supplemented on the basis of commentaries. Therefore, this maṇḍala may be closer to the original than V-10. In the Hahn Foundation handscroll, this maṇḍala lacks seats for Khecarī and Bhūcarī, and they have been added with reference to other examples. The colour scheme of the courtyard is that of the Highest Yoga tantras centred on Akṣobhya (Type E).

12. Fifteen-deity Kurukullā-maṇḍala

Pattern: 19. Eight-petalled lotus;
Colour scheme:
Highest Yoga tantras
centred on Amitābha

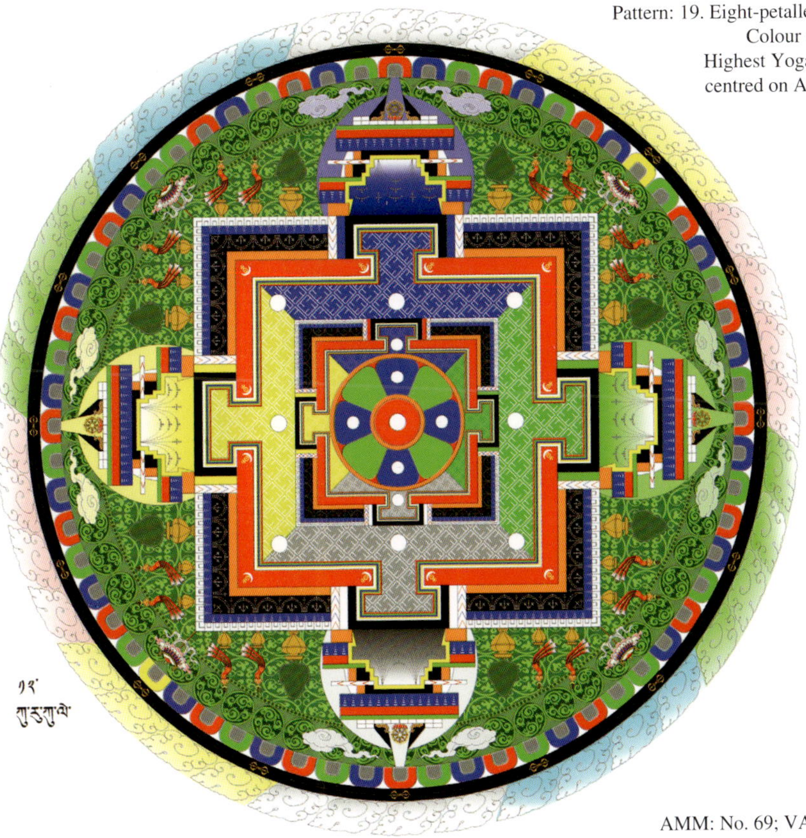

༡༢་
ཀུ་རུ་ཀུ་ལེ་

AMM: No. 69; VA: No. 6c

Kurukullā, also known as Red Tārā, is a female deity invoked in rites of attraction (*vaśīkaraṇa*) for winning the love of members of the opposite sex and superiors. The *Vajrāvalī* explains that if one changes the main deity of the fifteen-deity Nairātmyā-maṇḍala (V-11) to one-headed and four-armed Kurukullā and changes the colour of all the deities to red, the resultant maṇḍala is this Kurukullā-maṇḍala. The *Abhisamayamuktāmalā*, on the other hand, describes a completely different maṇḍala (No. 69), consisting of thirteen deities, with the main deity in the centre of a four-petalled lotus, the four Buddha-mothers on the four lotus petals in the four cardinal directions, the four inner offering goddesses Lāsyā, Mālā, Gītā and Nṛtyā in the four corners, and the four female gatekeepers Aṅkuśī, Pāśī, Sphoṭā and Ghaṇṭā in the four gates. It is not clear which form of this maṇḍala the Hahn Foundation handscroll depicts. However, it seems to have been executed with reference to the *Vajrāvalī* since its form is close to the fifteen-deity Nairātmyā-maṇḍala (V-11). The colour scheme of the courtyard is that of the Highest Yoga tantras centred on Amitābha (Type F), with the main deity having been changed from Akṣobhya to Amitābha. This is because Kurukullā, red in colour, belongs to the Lotus family presided over by Amitābha.

13. Nineteen-deity Vajratārā-maṇḍala

Pattern: 20. Eight-petalled lotus;
Colour scheme:
Highest Yoga tantras
centred on Ratnasambhava

༡༣
རྡོ་རྗེ་སྒྲོལ་མ་

AMM: No. 68; VA: No. 16

Tārā is a beautiful female bodhisattva who was born from the eye pupils (*tārā*) of Avalokiteśvara, and her cult became popular during the time of Esoteric Buddhism, as a result of which she came to be counted as one of the four Buddha-mothers. Vajratārā is one of the esoteric forms of Tārā. Her maṇḍala takes the form of an eight-petalled lotus, and four-headed and eight-armed Vajratārā, golden in colour, is depicted on the pericarp of the lotus. On the lotus petals in the four cardinal directions are four forms of Tārā—Puṣpatārā (east), Dhūpatārā (south), Dīpatārā (west) and Gandhatārā (north)—and in the four intermediate directions are the symbols of the four Buddhas, i.e., a wheel (southeast), a vajra (southwest), a lotus (northwest) and a sword (northeast). In the four gates are the four female gatekeepers Vajrāṅkuśī, Vajrapāśī, Vajrasphoṭā and Vajraghaṇṭā, while Uṣṇīṣavijayā and Sumbhā are at the top and bottom respectively. In the four corners of the courtyard are the symbols of the four Buddha-mothers, i.e., a vessel containing *bodhicitta*, Mount Meru, a hearth and a large banner. The Hahn Foundation handscroll depicts nineteen seats for deities (omitting the deities at the top and bottom), including their symbols, although the *Abhisamayamuktāmālā* gives the number of deities as eleven. The colour scheme of the courtyard is that of the Highest Yoga tantras centred on Ratnasambhava (Type G), with the main deity having been changed from Akṣobhya to Ratnasambhava. This is because Vajratārā, golden in colour, belongs to the Jewel family presided over by Ratnasambhava.

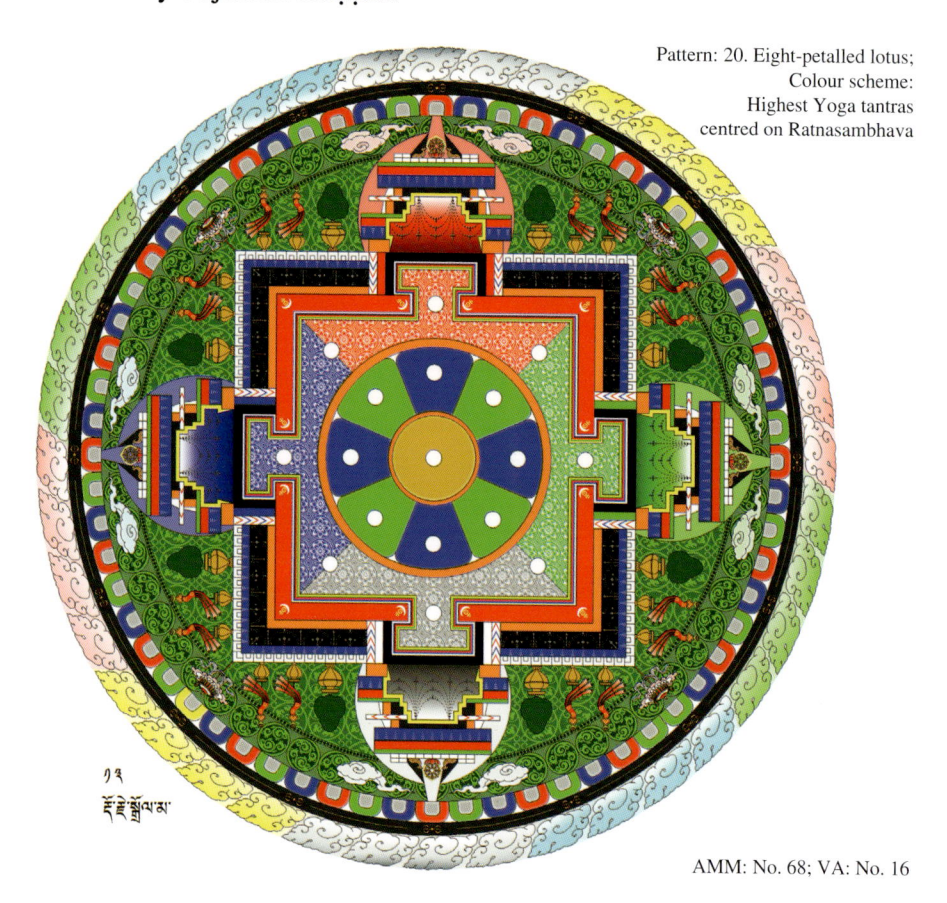

14. Seventeen-deity Garbha-Hevajra-maṇḍala

Pattern: 19. Eight-petalled lotus;
Colour scheme:
Highest Yoga tantras
centred on Akṣobhya

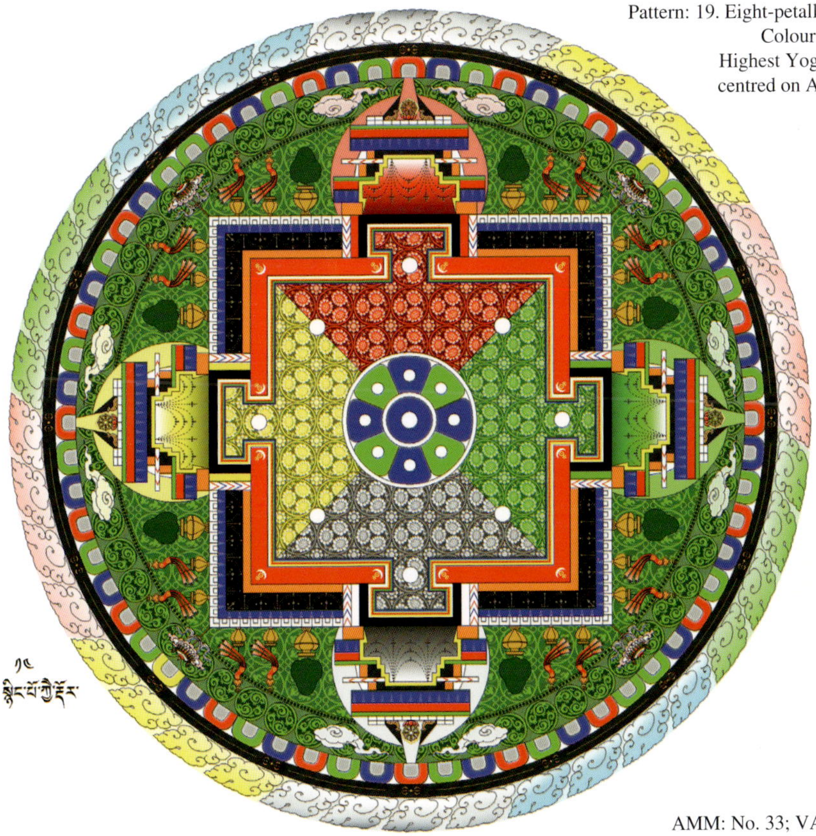

༡༨
སྙིང་པོ་ཀྱི་རྡོར་

AMM: No. 33; VA: No. 5a

Among the maṇḍalas of Hevajra, a representative tutelary deity of the Mother tantras, four nine-deity maṇḍalas (V-5~8) have already been described. The next four maṇḍalas are expounded in the *Saṃpuṭa-tantra*. The first, a seventeen-deity Garbha-Hevajra-maṇḍala, takes the form of an eight-petalled lotus, with eight-headed and sixteen-armed Hevajra and his one-headed and two-armed consort Nairātmyā depicted on the pericarp of the lotus. On the eight lotus petals are the same eight goddesses as appear in V-5: Gaurī (east), Caurī (south), Vetālī (west), Ghasmarī (north), Pukkasī (northeast), Śabarī (southeast), Caṇḍālī (southwest) and Ḍombī (northwest). In the four gates are four animal-headed female gatekeepers—Hayāsyā (east), Śūkarāsyā (south), Śvānāsyā (west) and Siṃhāsyā (north)—and in the four corners of the courtyard are the four goddesses of musical instruments, i.e., Vaṃśā (northeast), Vīṇā (southeast), Mukundā (southwest) and Murajā (northwest). The colour scheme of the courtyard is that of the Highest Yoga tantras centred on Akṣobhya (Type E).

15. Seventeen-deity Citta-Hevajra-maṇḍala

Pattern: 19. Eight-petalled lotus;
Colour scheme:
Highest Yoga tantras
centred on Akṣobhya

༡༥་

ཐུགས་ཀྱི་རྡོར་

AMM: No. 34; VA: No. 5b

This is the second of the four kinds of Hevajra-maṇḍala expounded in the *Saṃpuṭa-tantra* and is called "Citta-Hevajra," or "Mind-Hevajra," because it is assigned to the mind among the three mysteries of body, speech and mind. It is a variant form of the seventeen-deity Garbha-Hevajra-maṇḍala (V-14) in which eight-headed, sixteen-armed and four-legged Hevajra has been replaced as the main deity by a form of Hevajra with three heads—blue (front), white (right) and red (left)—and six arms. He is embracing his consort Vajraśṛṅkhalā and holds a vajra and a bell in his main right and left hands respectively. The *Niṣpannayogāvalī* states that in the three maṇḍalas (V-15~17) the eight goddesses surrounding the main deity, starting with Gaurī, should be changed to Vajraraudrī (east), Vajrabimbā (south), Rāgavajrā (west), Vajrasaumyā (north), Vajrayakṣī (northeast), Vajraḍākinī (southeast), Śabdavajrā (southwest) and Pṛthivīvajrā (northwest). The *Abhisamayamuktāmālā,* on the other hand, states that the attendant goddesses are the same as in the seventeen-deity Garbha-Hevajra-maṇḍala. The colour scheme of the courtyard is that of the Highest Yoga tantras centred on Akṣobhya (Type E).

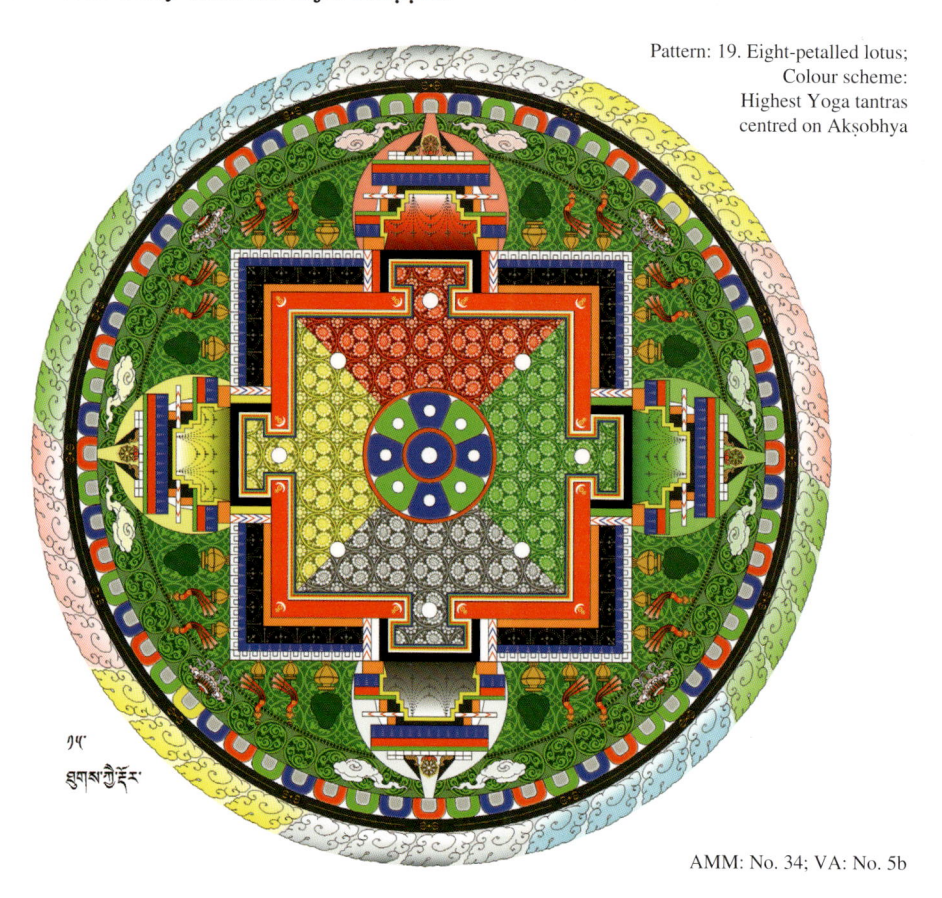

16. Seventeen-deity Vāk-Hevajra-maṇḍala

Pattern: 19. Eight-petalled lotus;
Colour scheme:
Highest Yoga tantras
centred on Akṣobhya

༡༦
གསུང་གྱི་རྡོར་

AMM: No. 34; VA: No. 5c

This is the third of the four kinds of Hevajra-maṇḍala expounded in the *Saṃpuṭa-tantra* and is called "Vāk-Hevajra," or "Speech-Hevajra," because it is assigned to speech among the three mysteries of body, speech and mind. It is a variant form of the seventeen-deity Garbha-Hevajra-maṇḍala (V-14) in which eight-headed, sixteen-armed and four-legged Hevajra has been replaced as the main deity by a one-headed and four-armed form of Hevajra who is embracing his consort Vajraśṛṅkhalā and holds a vajra and a bell in his main right and left hands respectively. According to the *Niṣpannayogāvalī,* the eight goddesses surrounding the main deity, starting with Gaurī, should be changed to the eight goddesses starting with Vajraraudrī. The *Abhisamayamuktāmālā,* on the other hand, states that the attendant goddesses are the same as in the seventeen-deity Garbha-Hevajra-maṇḍala. As in V-15, the colour scheme of the courtyard is that of the Highest Yoga tantras centred on Akṣobhya (Type E).

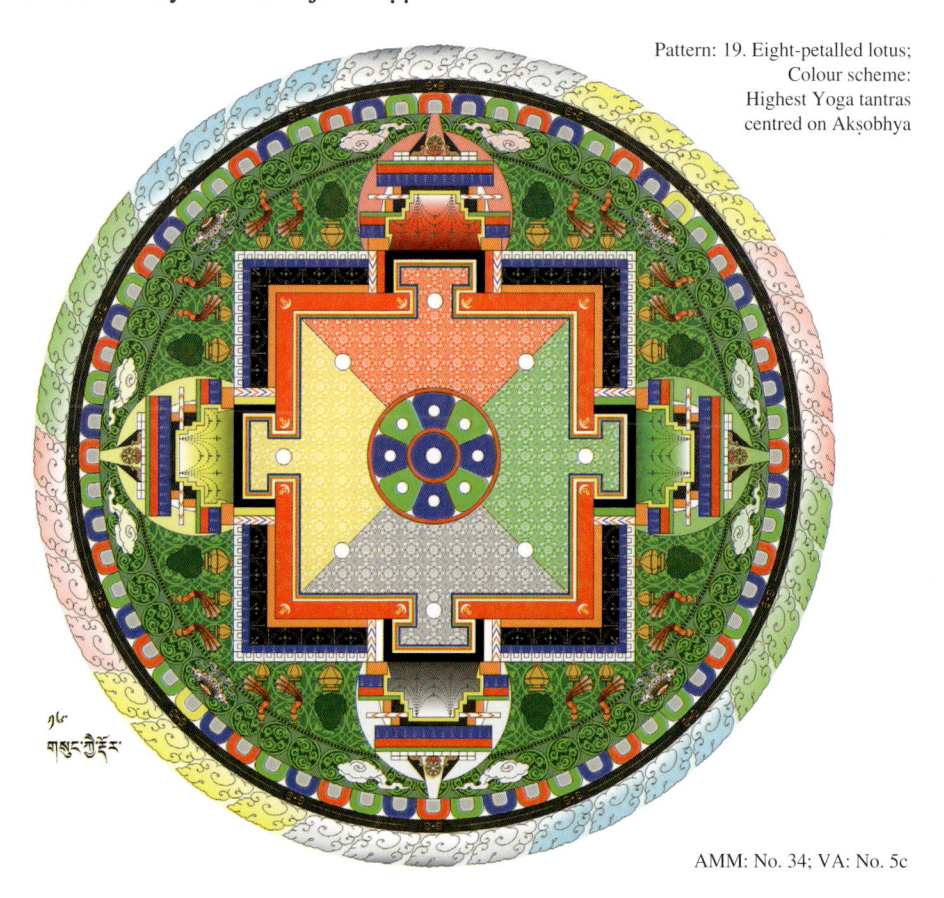

17. Seventeen-deity Kāya-Hevajra-maṇḍala

Pattern: 19. Eight-petalled lotus;
Colour scheme:
Highest Yoga tantras
centred on Akṣobhya

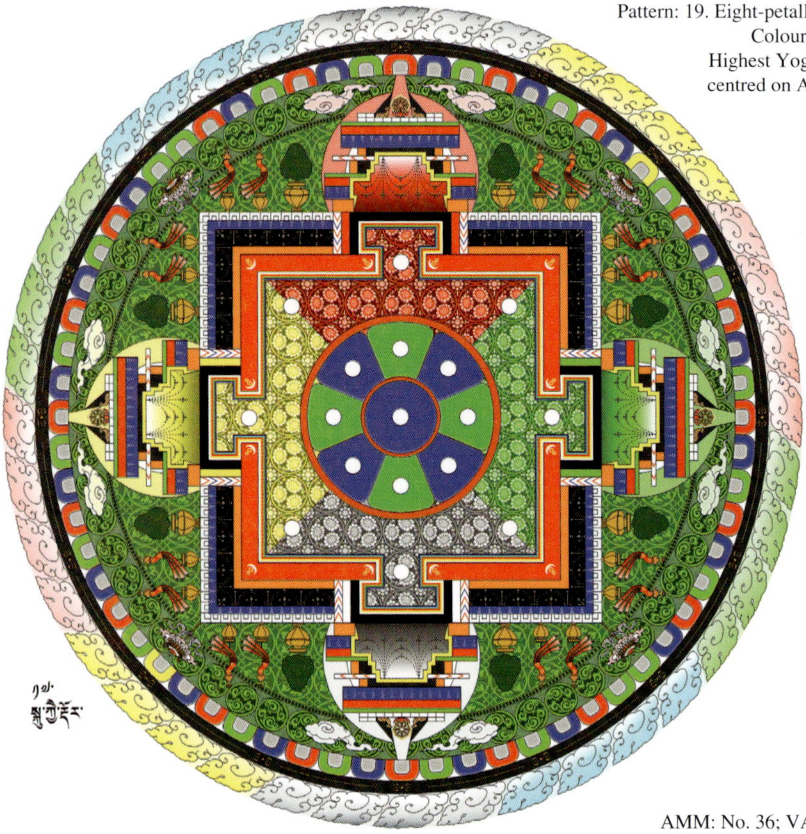

AMM: No. 36; VA: No. 5d

This is the fourth of the four kinds of Hevajra-maṇḍala expounded in the *Saṃpuṭa-tantra* and is called "Kāya-Hevajra," or "Body-Hevajra," because it is assigned to the body among the three mysteries of body, speech and mind. It is a variant form of the seventeen-deity Garbha-Hevajra-maṇḍala (V-14) in which eight-headed, sixteen-armed and four-legged Hevajra has been replaced as the main deity by a one-headed and two-armed form of Hevajra who is embracing his consort Nairātmyā and holds a vajra and a *kapāla* in his right and left hands respectively. According to the *Niṣpannayogāvalī,* the eight goddesses surrounding the main deity, starting with Gaurī, should be changed to the eight goddesses starting with Vajraraudrī. The *Abhisamayamuktāmālā,* on the other hand, states that the attendant goddesses are the same as in the seventeen-deity Garbha-Hevajra-maṇḍala. As in V-15, the colour scheme of the courtyard is that of the Highest Yoga tantras centred on Akṣobhya (Type E).

18. Thirty-seven-deity Saṃvara-Vajrasattva-maṇḍala

Pattern: 14. Nine-panel grid + eight-petalled lotus + eight-spoked wheel; Colour scheme: Highest Yoga tantras centred on Akṣobhya

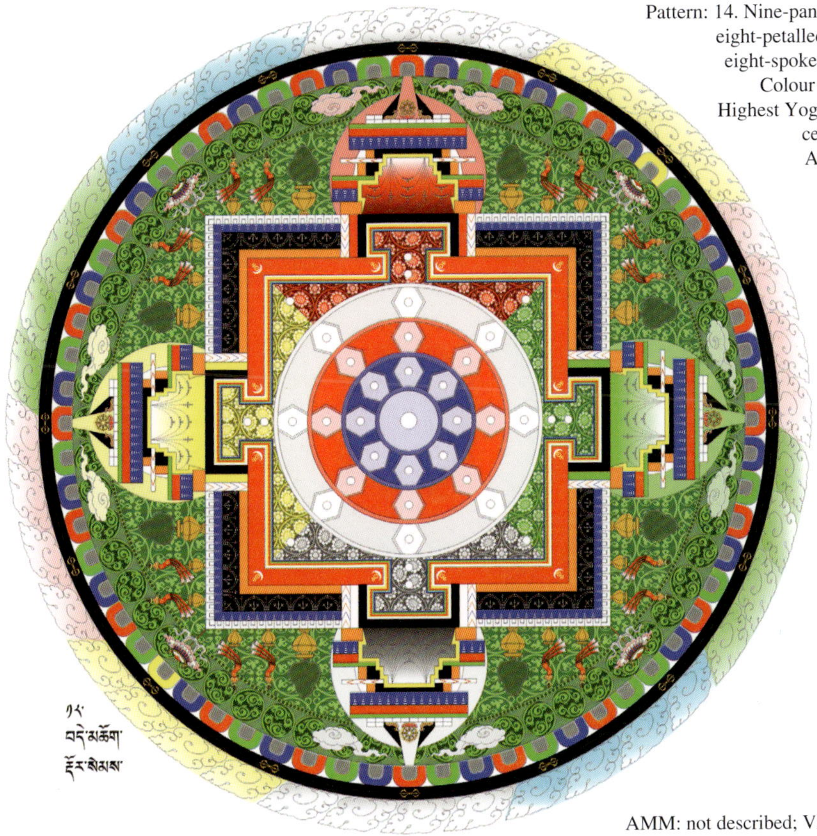

༡༨་
བདེ་མཆོག་
རྡོར་སེམས་

AMM: not described; VA: No. 3

Like the above four kinds of Hevajra-maṇḍala, this maṇḍala is also expounded in the *Saṃpuṭa-tantra*. According to *Roṅ tha's Iconometry*, this maṇḍala has a triple structure consisting, from the centre outwards, of a nine-panel grid, an eight-petalled lotus and an eight-spoked wheel. In the centre of the nine-panel grid the main deity Vajrasattva is depicted, while the five Buddhas Śāśvata (a.k.a. Vairocana; east), Ratnasambhava (south), Amitābha (west) and Amoghasiddhi (north) are arranged in the four cardinal directions and the four Buddha-mothers Locanā (northeast), Māmakī (southeast), Pāṇḍarā (southwest) and Tārā (northwest) in the intermediate directions around the main deity. In the second circle are the same eight goddesses, starting with Vajraraudrī, as appear in the Citta-Hevajra-maṇḍala (V-15). In the third circle are the four offering goddesses of the *Paramādya-tantra*—Hāsyā, Lāsyā, Gītā and Nṛtyā—in the four cardinal directions and the four goddesses of musical instruments starting with Vaṃśā in the intermediate directions. Outside the triple eight-spoked wheel are the four outer offering goddesses Puṣpā, Dhūpā, Dīpā and Gandhā in the intermediate directions and the four goddesses Ādarśā, Rasā, Sparśā and Dharmā in the four cardinal directions. The *Abhisamayamuktāmālā* does not describe this maṇḍala. The Hahn Foundation handscroll depicts this maṇḍala in the form of a triple eight-spoked wheel, like the sixty-two-deity Cakrasaṃvara-maṇḍala (V-19) from which the central eight-petalled lotus has been removed. The colour scheme of the courtyard is that of the Highest Yoga tantras centred on Akṣobhya (Type E).

19. Sixty-two-deity Cakrasaṃvara-maṇḍala

Pattern: 13. Triple eight-spoked wheel;
Colour scheme: Highest Yoga tantras centred on Akṣobhya

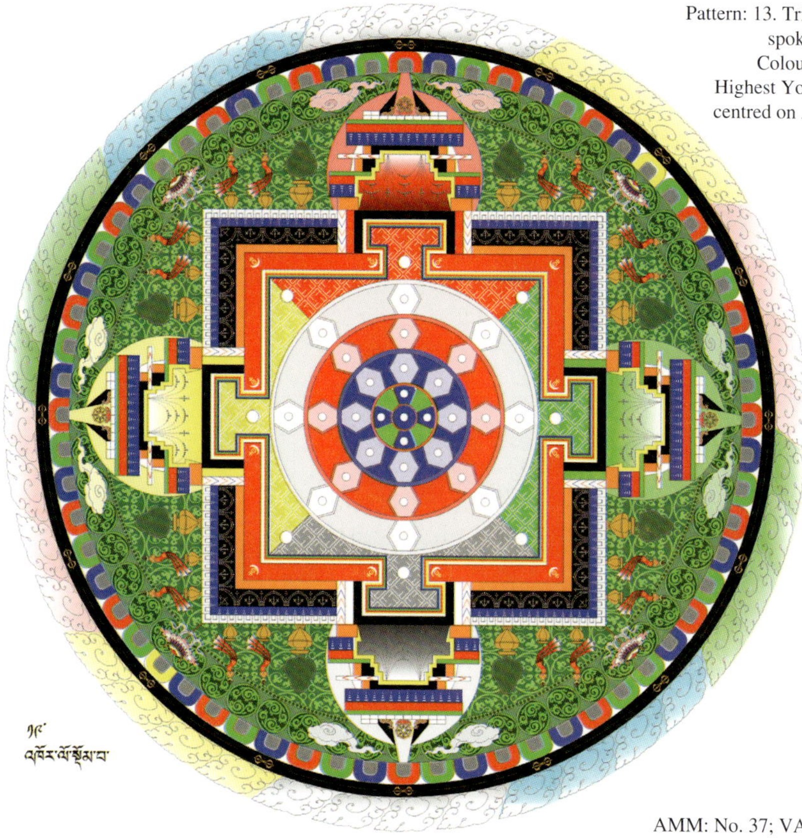

AMM: No. 37; VA: No. 12a

The *Saṃvara-tantra*, along with the *Hevajra-tantra*, is a representative Mother tantra of the Highest Yoga tantras. This maṇḍala represents the basic style of the various maṇḍalas of the Saṃvara cycle, among which this maṇḍala is the most popular. It takes the form of a triple eight-spoked wheel surrounding an eight-petalled lotus. The eight-petalled lotus, the three eight-spoked wheels and the outer square are called the wheel of great bliss (*mahāsukha-cakra*), the wheel of the mind (*citta-cakra*), the wheel of speech (*vāk-cakra*), the wheel of the body (*kāya-cakra*) and the wheel of the pledge (*samaya-cakra*) respectively. In the centre of the wheel of great bliss, the main deity Saṃvara and his consort Vajravārāhī are depicted. On the lotus petals in the cardinal directions are the four goddesses Ḍākinī (east), Lāmā (north), Khaṇḍarohā (west) and Rūpiṇī (south), while *kapāla*s are depicted on the four lotus petals in the intermediate directions. The eight-petalled lotus is surrounded by a triple eight-spoked wheel with eight couples arranged in the cardinal and intermediate directions of each wheel. Thus the total number of couples on the wheels of the three mysteries is twenty-four. The outermost square is called the wheel of the pledge, and in the four gates are four animal-headed female gatekeepers—Kākāsyā (east), Ulūkāsyā (north), Śvānāsyā (west) and Śūkarāsyā (south)—while the four goddesses Yamaḍāḍhī (southeast), Yamadūtī (southwest), Yamadaṃṣṭrī (northwest) and Yamamathanī (northeast) are arranged in the four corners of the courtyard. The colour scheme of the courtyard is that of the Highest Yoga tantras centred on Akṣobhya (Type E).

20. Sixty-two-deity maṇḍala of two-armed Saṃvara

Pattern: 13. Triple eight-spoked wheel;
Colour scheme:
Highest Yoga tantras
centred on Akṣobhya

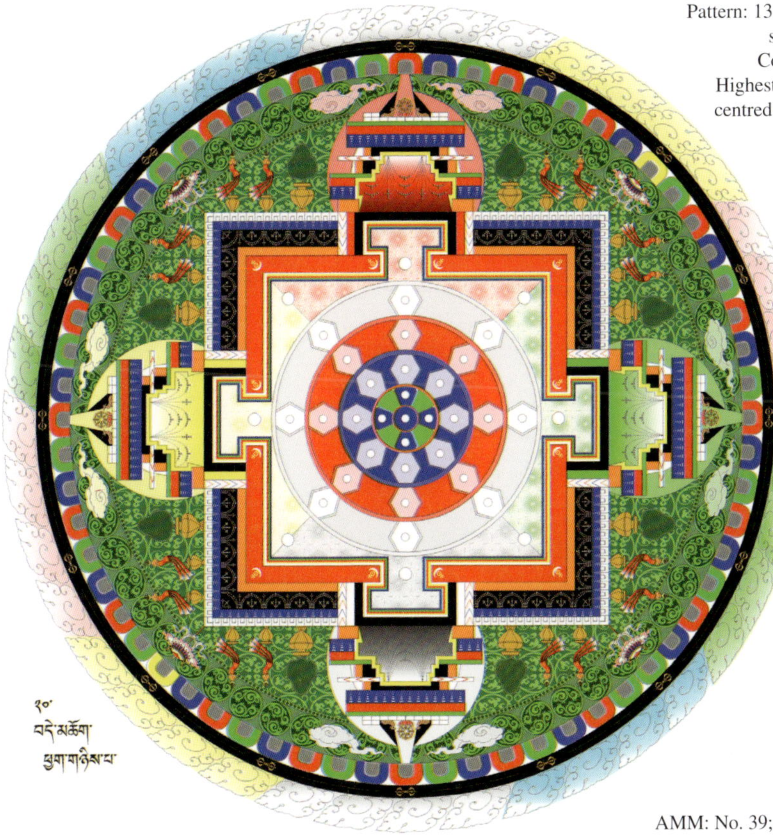

༢༠་
བདེ་མཆོག་
ཕྱག་གཉིས་པ་

AMM: No. 39; VA: No. 12b

This maṇḍala is a variant form of the sixty-two-deity Cakrasaṃvara-maṇḍala (V-19) in which four-headed and twelve-armed Saṃvara has been replaced as the main deity by a one-headed and two-armed form of Saṃvara. It is described in the *Niṣpannayogāvalī*. In this case, all the attendant deities from Ḍākinī to Yamamathanī are also one-headed and two-armed. The main deity and heroes (male deities) on the wheels of the three mysteries hold a vajra in their right hand and a vajra-bell in their left hand. The four goddesses starting with Ḍākinī on the wheel of great bliss and the eight goddesses on the wheel of the pledge hold a *ḍamaru* (hand drum) in their right hand and a *kapāla* in their left hand and have a *khaṭvāṅga* (staff with a skull on the top) leaning against their shoulder. As in V-19, the colour scheme of the courtyard is that of the Highest Yoga tantras centred on Akṣobhya (Type E).

21. Sixty-two-deity maṇḍala of Yellow Saṃvara

Pattern: 13. Triple eight-spoked wheel;
Colour scheme: Highest Yoga tantras centred on Akṣobhya

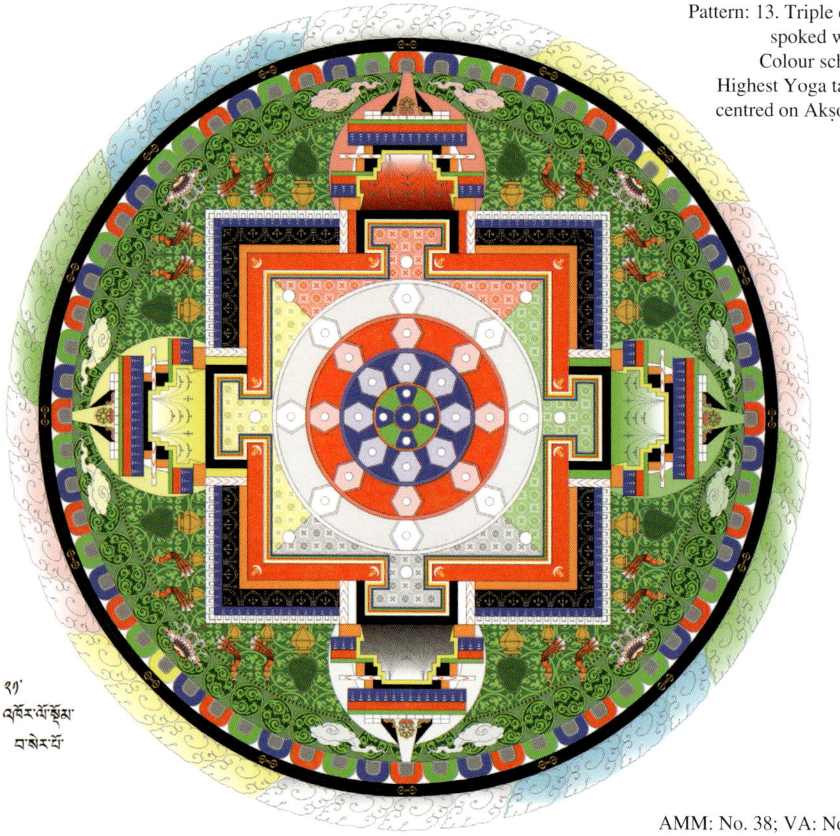

༢༡་
འཁོར་ལོ་སྡོམ་
པ་སེར་པོ་

AMM: No. 38; VA: No. 12c

This maṇḍala is a variant form of the sixty-two-deity maṇḍala of two-armed Saṃvara (V-20) in which two-armed Blue Saṃvara has been replaced as the main deity by two-armed Saṃvara and his consort Vajravārāhī, both golden in colour. It is described in the *Niṣpannayogāvalī*, according to which the four goddeses starting with Ḍākinī on the wheel of great bliss are golden in colour, the heroes (male deities) on the wheel of the mind are blue and the heroines (female deities) white, the heroes on the wheel of speech are red and the *ḍākinī*s (female deities) blue, and the heroes on the wheel of the body are white and the goddesses red. The Hahn Foundation handscroll does not show these features since it indicates the seats for the deities by means of small white circles. As in V-19, the colour scheme of the courtyard is that of the Highest Yoga tantras centred on Akṣobhya (Type E).

22. Thirty-seven-deity maṇḍala of Red Vajravārāhī

Pattern: 13. Triple eight-spoked wheel;
Colour scheme: Highest Yoga tantras centred on Akṣobhya

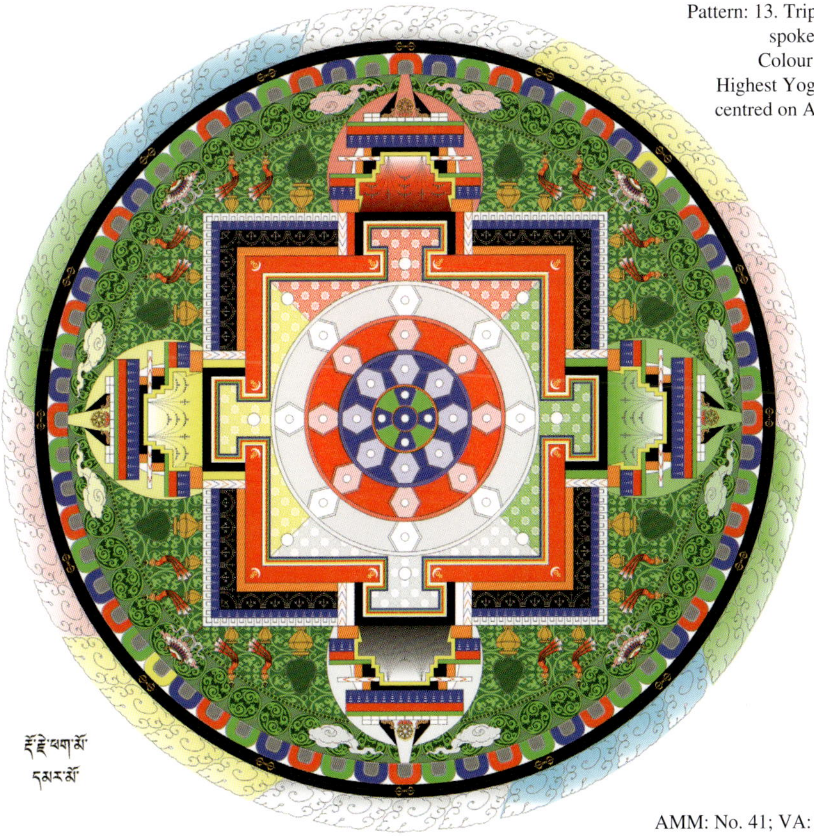

AMM: No. 41; VA: No. 12d

This maṇḍala is a variant form of the sixty-two-deity Cakrasaṃvara-maṇḍala (V-19), the basic style of maṇḍalas in the Saṃvara-cycle, in which Saṃvara accompanied by his consort has been replaced as the main deity by his consort Vajravārāhī, red in colour. In the Saṃvara literature there exists in addition to the "father cycle" (*yab 'khor*) centred on the male Saṃvara a "mother cycle" (*yum 'khor*) centred on his consort Vajravārāhī. In maṇḍalas of the mother cycle, heroes (male deities) do not appear and only heroines (female deities) are depicted on the wheels of the three mysteries. Thus, the total number of deities, as explained in the *Abhisamayamuktāmālā*, is thirty-seven. As in V-19, the colour scheme of the courtyard is that of the Highest Yoga tantras centred on Akṣobhya (Type E).

23. Thirty-seven-deity maṇḍala of Blue Vajravārāhī

Pattern: 13. Triple eight-spoked wheel;
Colour scheme: Highest Yoga tantras centred on Akṣobhya

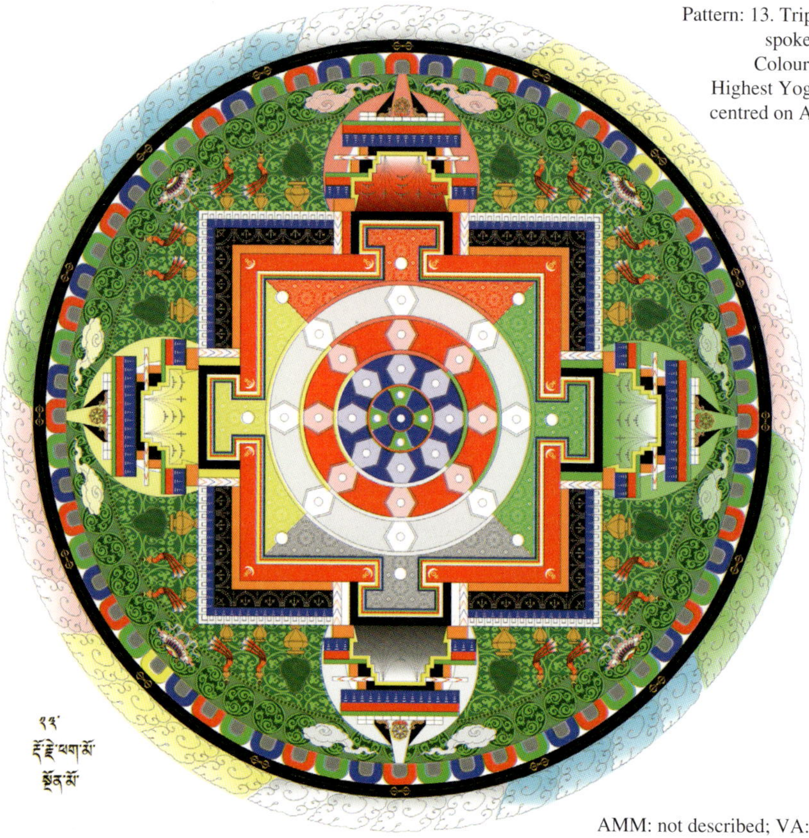

༢༣་
རྡོ་རྗེ་ཕག་མོ་
སྔོན་མོ་

AMM: not described; VA: No. 12e

This maṇḍala is a variant form of the sixty-two-deity Cakrasaṃvara-maṇḍala (V-19), the basic style of maṇḍalas in the Saṃvara-cycle, in which Saṃvara accompanied by his consort has been replaced as the main deity by his consort Vajravārāhī, blue in colour. As is usual in the Saṃvara mother cycle, heroes do not appear on the wheels of the three mysteries, and only heroines are depicted. This maṇḍala is not described in the *Abhisamayamuktāmālā*. As in the case of the maṇḍala of Red Vajravārāhī (V-22), the total number of deities is thirty-seven. As in V-19, the colour scheme of the courtyard is that of the Highest Yoga tantras centred on Akṣobhya (Type E).

24. Thirty-seven-deity maṇḍala of Yellow Vajravārāhī

Pattern: 13. Triple eight-spoked wheel;
Colour scheme: Highest Yoga tantras centred on Akṣobhya

༢༨་
རྡོ་རྗེ་ཕག་མོ་
སེར་མོ་

AMM: not described; VA: No. 12f

This maṇḍala is a variant form of the sixty-two-deity maṇḍala of Yellow Saṃvara (V-21) in which Yellow Saṃvara accompanied by his consort has been replaced as the main deity by his consort Vajravārāhī, golden in colour. As is usual in the Saṃvara mother cycle, heroes do not appear on the wheels of the three mysteries, and only heroines are depicted. This maṇḍala is not described in the *Abhisamayamuktāmālā*. As in the case of the maṇḍala of Red Vajravārāhī (V-22), the total number of deities is thirty-seven. As in V-19, the colour scheme of the courtyard is that of the Highest Yoga tantras centred on Akṣobhya (Type E).

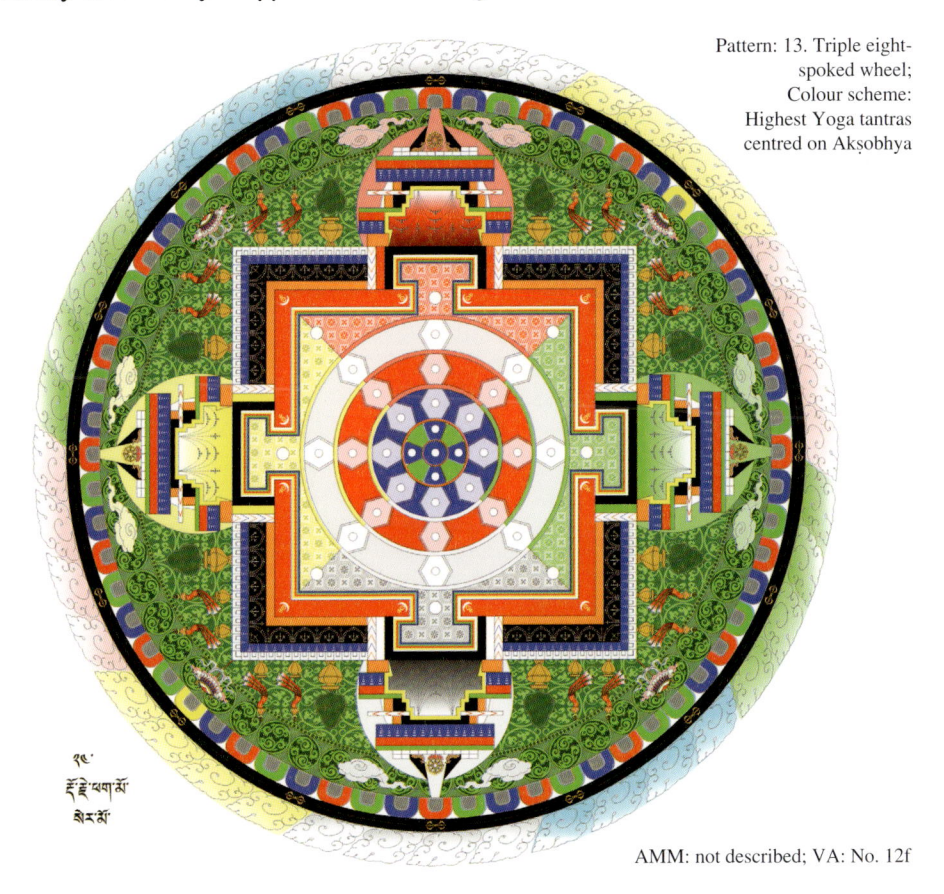

25. Eleven-deity Krodhahūṃkāra-maṇḍala

Pattern: 7. Eleven eight-petalled lotuses; Colour scheme: Highest Yoga tantras centred on Akṣobhya

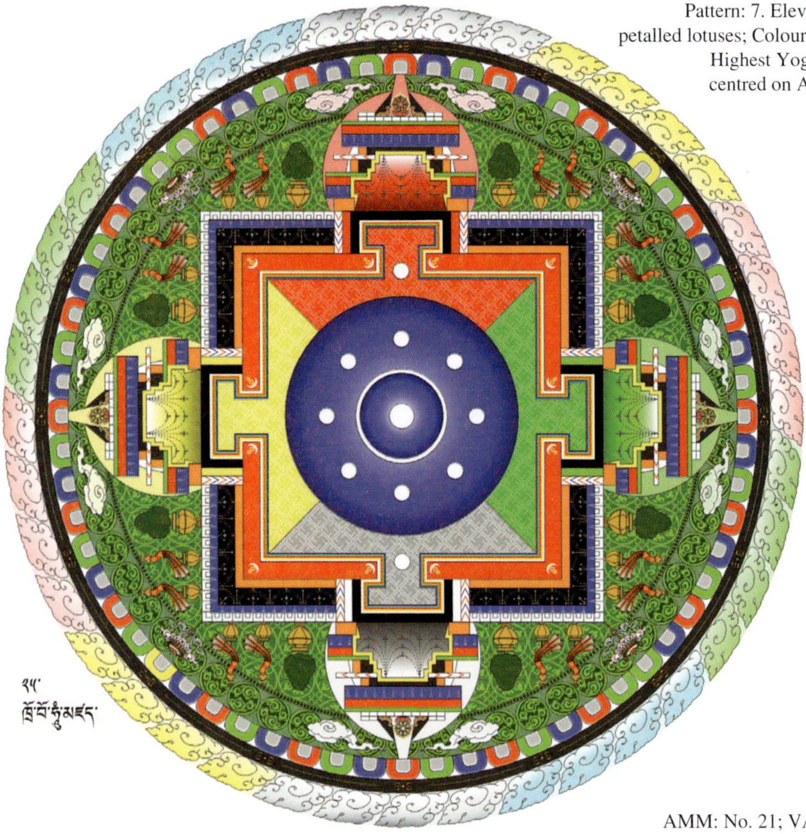

༢༥་
ཁྲོ་བོ་ཧཱུྃ་མཛད་

AMM: No. 21; VA: No. 11

According to *Roṅ tha's Iconometry*, this maṇḍala has eleven eight-petalled lotuses in its courtyard and depicts the main deity Vajrahūṃkāra on the central lotus, while ten wrathful deities, the protectors of the ten directions, are arranged on ten eight-petalled lotuses surrounding the main deity, although Uṣṇīṣacakravartin at the top and Vajrapātāla at the bottom are actually depicted in the east (top) and west (bottom) respectively. The colour scheme of the courtyard is that of the Highest Yoga tantras centred on Akṣobhya (Type E). As the textual source for this maṇḍala, *Roṅ tha's Iconometry* points to the *Guhyasamāja-tantra*, while lCaṅ skya II (1642–1714) gives the *Abhidhānottara-tantra*. However, this maṇḍala was not very popular in Tibet. The Hahn Foundation handscroll does not depict the eleven eight-petalled lotuses prescribed in *Roṅ tha's Iconometry* and instead shows eight wrathful deities in the eight directions on a large blue disc. Although the seats for the two wrathful deities at the top and bottom are not depicted in the original, they have been added with reference to other examples. In the Hahn Foundation collection, there is another example of this maṇḍala, finely executed and going back to the fourteenth century, which seems not to be an independent work, but to have formed part of a *Vajrāvalī* set.

26. Ṣaṭcakravartin-maṇḍala

Pattern: Composite type;
Colour scheme:
Highest Yoga tantras
centred on Akṣobhya

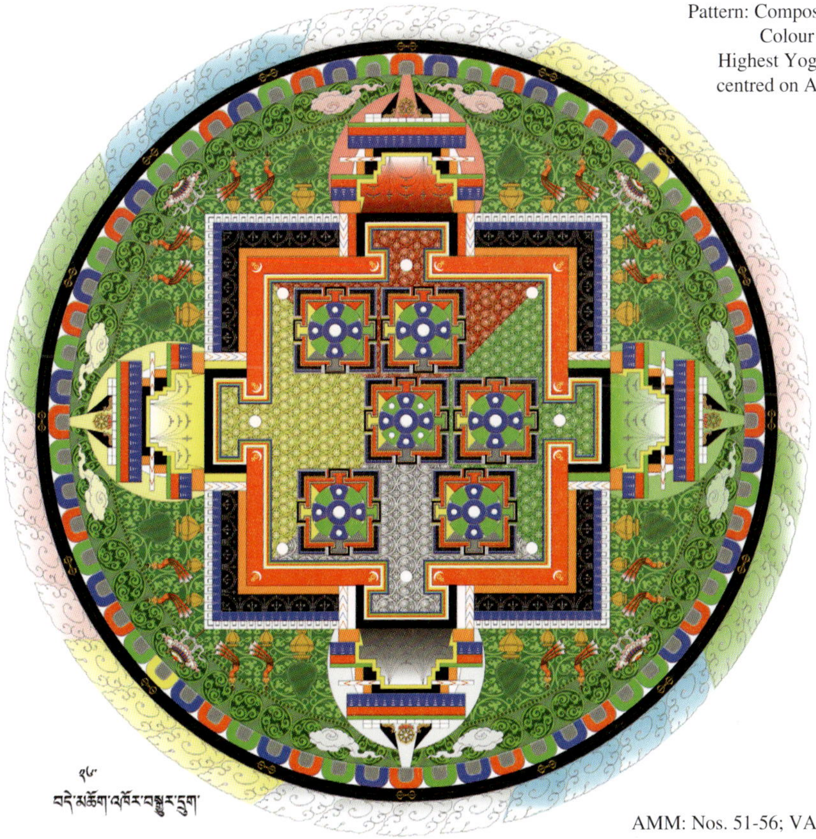

༢༦
བདེ་མཆོག་འཁོར་བསྒྱུར་དྲུག་

AMM: Nos. 51-56; VA: No. 25

Ṣaṭcakravartin means "six universal rulers," and this maṇḍala is expounded in the *Abhidhānottara-tantra*, an *uttaratantra* (continuation tantra) of the Saṃvara cycle. It is of a composite type, consisting of six pavilions of Jñānaḍāka (centre), Buddhaḍāka (east), Ratnaḍāka (south), Padmaḍāka (southwest), Vajraḍāka (northwest) and Viśvaḍāka (north). The *Abhisamayamuktāmālā* treats these maṇḍalas as six independent maṇḍalas (Nos. 51-56). In the four intermediate directions of the central pavilion are the four goddesses Ḍākinī, Lāmā, Khaṇḍarohā and Rūpinī, the same four goddesses as are depicted on the wheel of great bliss in the sixty-two-deity Cakrasaṃvara-maṇḍala (V-19). The twenty-four couples depicted on the wheels of the three mysteries, on the other hand, are assigned to the pavilions of the six universal rulers or *ḍāka*s. In the four gates of the outer pavilion are the four animal-headed female gatekeepers starting with Kākāsyā, and in the four corners of the outer pavilion are the four wrathful goddesses starting with Yamaḍāḍhī. As in other maṇḍalas of the Saṃvara cycle, the colour scheme of the courtyard is that of the Highest Yoga tantras centred on Akṣobhya (Type E).

27. Twenty-one-deity Vajrāmṛta-maṇḍala

Pattern:19. Eight-petalled lotus;
Colour scheme:
Highest Yoga tantras
centred on Akṣobhya

༢༧་

རྡོ་རྗེ་བདུད་རྩི་

AMM: not described; VA: No. 7a

The following four maṇḍalas (V-27~30), collectively called "four kinds of Vajrāmṛta" in ritual manuals, correspond to the Vajrāmṛta-maṇḍala expounded in the *Vajrāmṛta-tantra* and its variant forms, none of which are explained in the *Abhisamayamuktāmālā*. This maṇḍala has an eight-petalled lotus in the centre, on the pericarp of which three-headed and six-armed Vajrāmṛta accompanied by his consort is depicted as the main deity. On the lotus petals in the eight directions are the eight female deities Saumyā (east), Saumyavadanā (south), Cāndrī (west), Śaśinī (north), Śaṣimaṇḍā (northeast), Śaśilekhā (southeast), Manojñā (southwest) and Manohrādanakarī (northwest). In the four intermediate directions of the outer square are the four inner offering goddesses Lāsyā, Mālā, Gītā and Nṛtyā, while in the four cardinal directions of the outer square are the four goddesses of musical instruments starting with Vaṃśā. In the four gates are the four gatekeepers Bhṛkuṭītaraṅga (east), Bhayabhīṣaṇa (south), Hayarūpa (west) and Gaṇanāyaka (north). Although Vajrāmṛta belongs to the Vajrasūrya clan, which corresponds to the Jewel family (Ratnakula) of the Father tantras, the colour scheme of the courtyard is that of the Highest Yoga tantras centred on Akṣobhya (Type E).

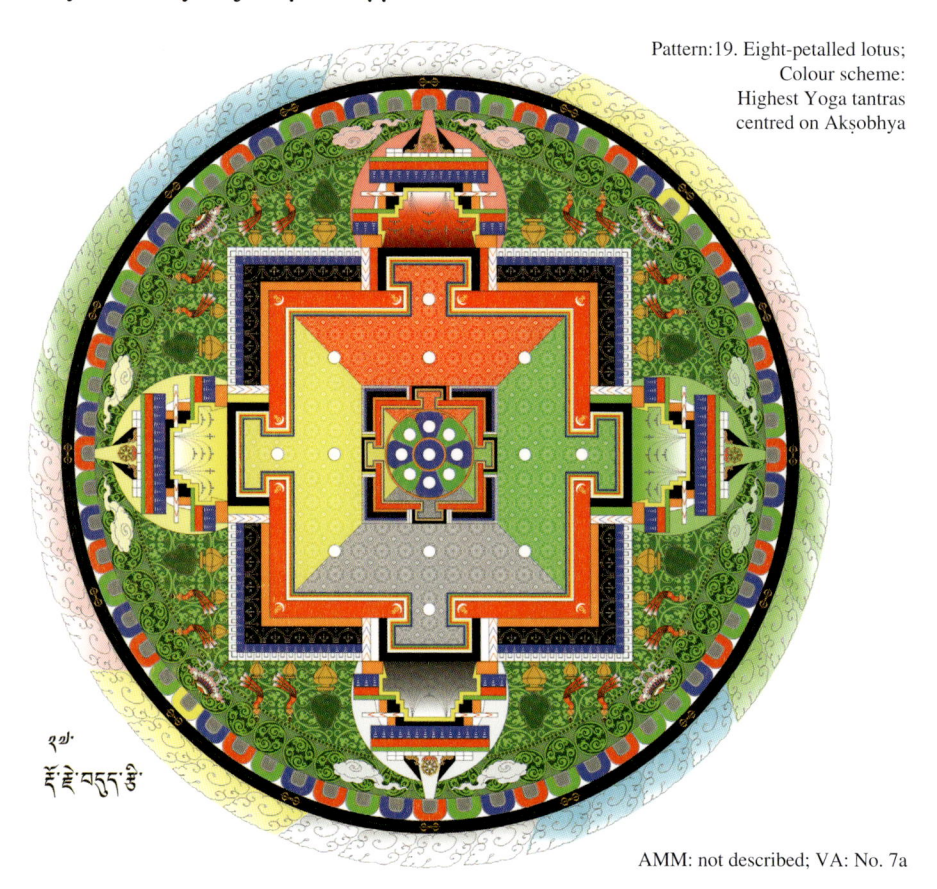

28. Twenty-nine-deity Vajrahūṃkāra-maṇḍala

Pattern: 19. Eight-petalled lotus;
Colour scheme:
Highest Yoga tantras
centred on Akṣobhya

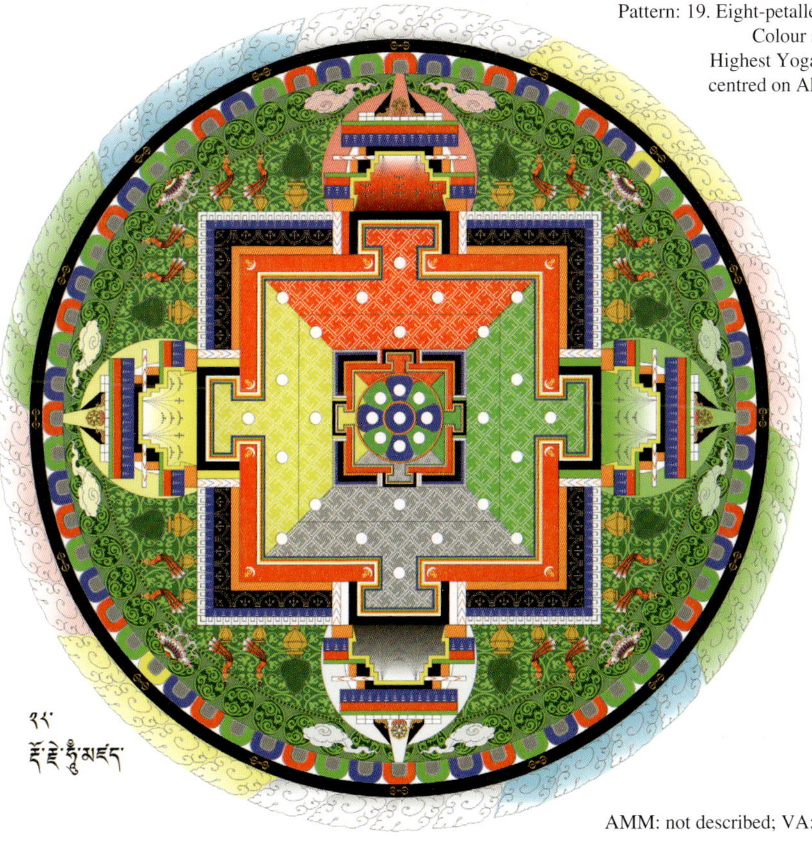

༢༨
རྡོ་རྗེ་ཧཱུྃ་མཛད་

AMM: not described; VA: No. 7b

As an example of a maṇḍala of Vajrahūṃkāra, the eleven-deity Krodhahūṃkāra-maṇḍala (V-25) has already been described. The present maṇḍala is a variant form of the twenty-one-deity Vajrāmṛta-maṇḍala (V-27). Neither the *Vajrāvalī* nor the *Niṣpannayogāvalī* give details of the three variations of the Vajrāmṛta-maṇḍala and state only that reference should be made to the *Vajrāmṛta-tantra*. This maṇḍala has an eight-petalled lotus in the centre, on the pericarp of which three-headed and six-armed Vajrahūṃkāra is depicted as the main deity. On the lotus petals in the four cardinal directions are the four female deities Vajragarbhā (east), Vajraśastrā (south), Sparśavajrā (west) and Kilikilā (north), and on the lotus petals in the four intermediate directions are four vases filled with *amṛta* (nectar). (In the Hahn Foundation handscroll these are indicated by means of small circles.) In addition, in the four cardinal directions of the outer pavilion (inside) are the four goddesses of musical instruments, i.e., Vaṃśā (east), Vīṇā (south), Mukundā (west) and Murajā (north); in the four intermediate directions are the four inner offering goddesses Lāsyā, Mālā, Gītā and Nṛtyā; in the surrounding strips of the outer pavilion are the eight great bodhisattvas; in the four corners of the outer pavilion are the four outer offering goddesses Puṣpā, Dhūpā, Dīpā and Gandhā; and in the four gates are the four female gatekeepers Aṅkuśī, Pāśī, Sphoṭā and Ghaṇṭā. The colour scheme of the courtyard is that of the Highest Yoga tantras centred on Akṣobhya (Type E).

29. Twenty-one-deity Vajraheruka-maṇḍala

Pattern: 19. Eight-petalled lotus;
Colour scheme:
Highest Yoga tantras
centred on Akṣobhya

༢༩་
རྡོ་རྗེ་ཁྲག་
འཐུང་

AMM: not described; VA: No. 7c

This is the second of the three variant forms of the twenty-one-deity Vajrāmṛta-maṇḍala (V-27). It has an eight-petalled lotus in the centre, with four-headed and eight-armed Vajraheruka on its pericarp as the main deity. On the lotus petals in the eight directions are eight goddesses: gTsigs chen ma (east), rNam gtsigs ma (south), gTum mo (west), gYuṅ mo (north), Ser skya ma (southeast), Ku li ni (southwest), Drag mo (northwest), and 'Jigs byed ma (northeast) (—their Sanskrit names are not given in the *Vajrāvalī* or *Niṣpannayogāvalī*). In the four cardinal directions of the surrounding strip are the four outer offering goddesses Puṣpā, Dhūpā, Dīpā and Gandhā; in the four intermediate directions are the four goddesses of musical instruments, i.e., Vīṇā (southeast), Vaṃśā (southwest), Mukundā (northwest) and Murajā (northeast); and in the four gates are the four gatekeepers Ba glaṅ sna (east), Glaṅ chen sna (south), Źal mdzes ma (west) and Źal sdug ma (north) (—their Sanskrit names are also not given in the *Vajrāvalī* or *Niṣpanna-yogāvalī*). The colour scheme of the courtyard is that of the Highest Yoga tantras centred on Akṣobhya (Type E).

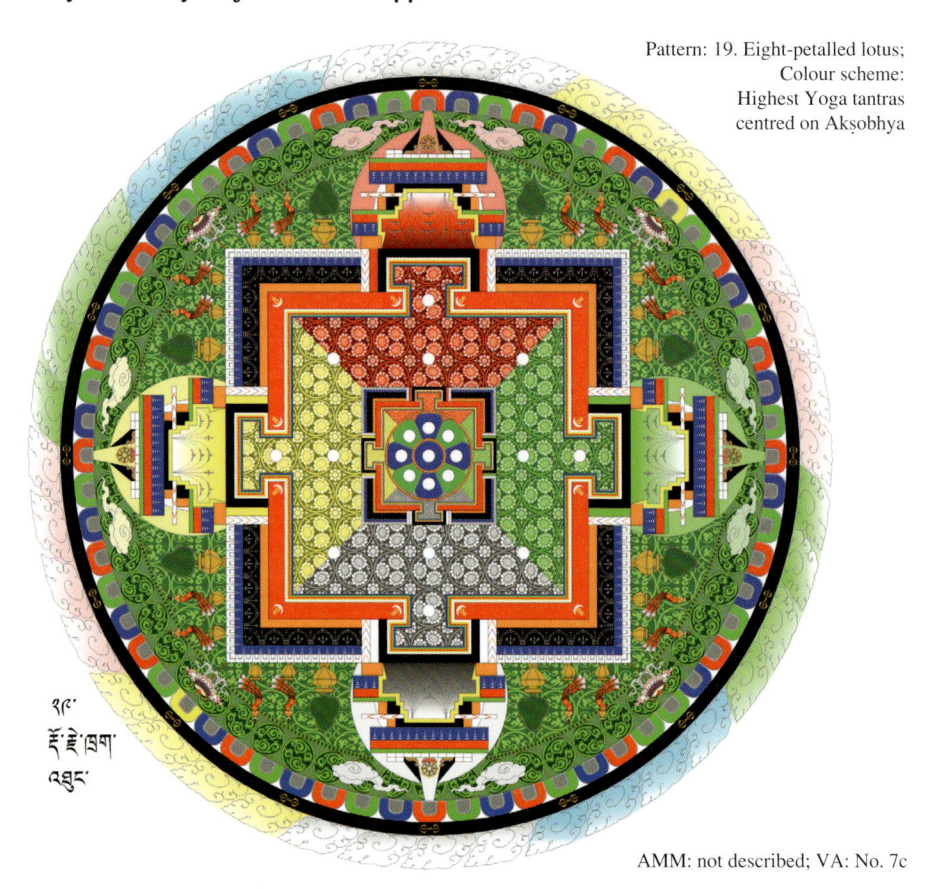

30. Thirteen-deity Amṛtakuṇḍalin-maṇḍala

Pattern: 19. Eight-petalled lotus;
Colour scheme:
Highest Yoga tantras
centred on Akṣobhya

AMM: not described; VA: No. 7d

This is the third of the three variant forms of the twenty-one-deity Vajrāmṛta-maṇḍala (V-27). It has an eight-petalled lotus in the centre, on the pericarp of which three-headed and six-armed Amṛtakuṇḍalin is depicted as the main deity. On the lotus petals in the eight directions are eight goddesses: rDo rje bdud rtsi ma (east), bDud rtsi źal ma (south), bDud rtsi'i lus can ma (west), bDud rtsi spyan ma (north), A me ya (southeast), gZugs bzag ma (southwest), mDzes pa'i gzugs can ma (northwest) and bDe sgrub ma (northeast) (—their Sanskrit names are not given in the *Vajrāvalī* or *Niṣpannayogāvalī*). In the four gates are the four female gatekeepers Aṅkuśī, Pāśī, Sphoṭā and Ghaṇṭā. Thus, the total number of deities is thirteen. The colour scheme of the courtyard is that of the Highest Yoga tantras centred on Akṣobhya (Type E).

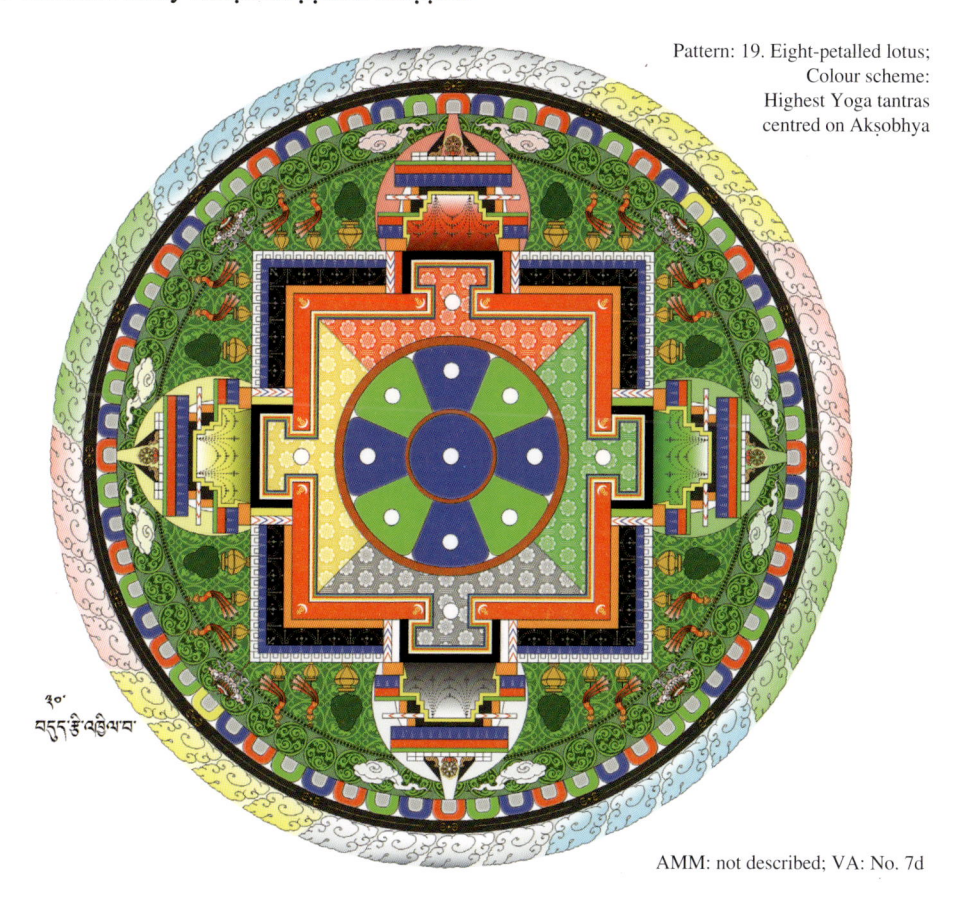

31. Twenty-five-deity Buddhakapāla-maṇḍala

Pattern: 13. Triple eight-spoked wheel; Colour scheme: Highest Yoga tantras centred on Akṣobhya

༣༡་
སངས་རྒྱས་
ཐོད་པ།

AMM: No. 66; VA: No. 13

This maṇḍala is based on the *Buddhakapāla-tantra*, one of the Mother tantras of the Highest Yoga tantras. *Roṅ tha's Iconometry* describes this maṇḍala as a triple eight-spoked wheel similar to the sixty-two-deity Cakrasaṃvara-maṇḍala (V-19). The Hahn Foundation handscroll depicts it in the form of a double eight-spoked wheel surrounding an eight-petalled lotus, and several other examples of this maṇḍala coincide with this depiction. On the pericarp of the eight-petalled lotus four-armed Buddhakapāla accompanied by his consort Citrasenā is depicted as the main deity. On the lotus petals in the four cardinal directions the four goddesses Sumālinī (east), Kapālinī (north), Bhīmā (west) and Sudurjayā (south) are arranged counterclockwise. The Hahn Foundation handscroll depicts small circles representing the seats for deities in the intermediate directions too. However, these circles are not the seats for deities, but *kapāla*s depicted on the lotus petals in the intermediate directions. On the first eight-spoked wheel surrounding the lotus are eight goddesses, starting with Śubhamekhalā, and on the second eight-spoked wheel are a further eight goddesses, starting with Tāriṇī. The four gates are occupied by the four female gatekeepers Sundarī (east), Vasundharā (north), Subhagā (west) and Priyadarśanā (south). The colour scheme of the courtyard is that of the Highest Yoga tantras centred on Akṣobhya (Type E).

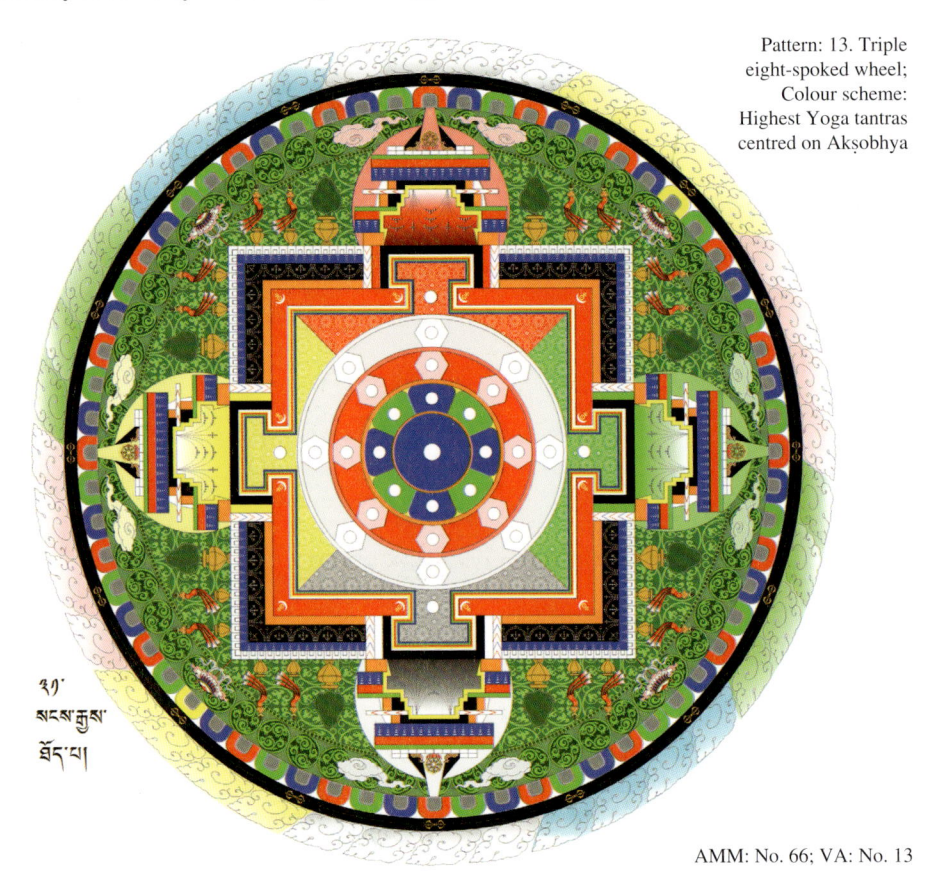

32. Nine-deity Buddhakapāla-maṇḍala

Pattern: 16. Eight petalled lotus;
Colour scheme:
special type

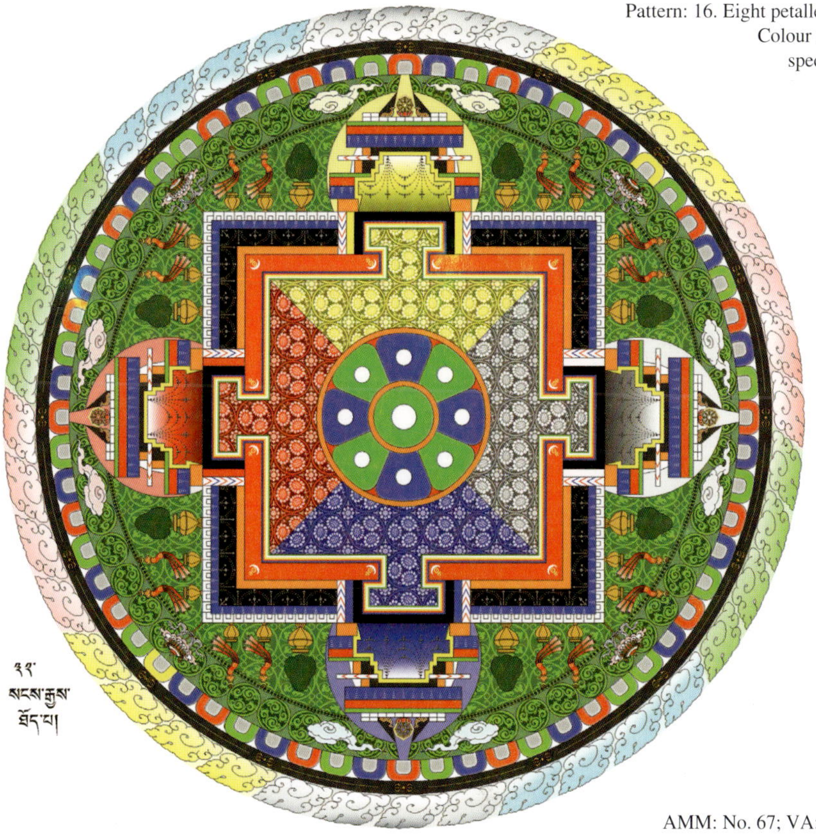

༣༢་
སངས་རྒྱས་
ཐོད་པ།

AMM: No. 67; VA: No. 10

Like the twenty-five-deity Buddhakapāla-maṇḍala (V-31), this maṇḍala is also based on the *Buddhakapāla-tantra.* However, its form and the arrangement of the deities are quite different. This maṇḍala takes the form of an eight-petalled lotus, on the pericarp of which four-armed Buddhakapāla without a consort is depicted as the main deity. On the lotus petals in the eight directions the eight goddesses Citrasenā (east), Kāminī (north), Pātālavāsinī (west), Saubhadrā (south), Śauṇḍinī (northeast), Bhūtinī (southeast), Caturbhujā (southwest) and Ākāśavāsinī (northwest) are arranged counterclockwise. The Hahn Foundation handscroll adopts an unusual colour scheme for the courtyard consisting of blue (east), white (north), yellow (west) and red (south). This is because, according to the *Niṣpannayogāvalī*, the four goddesses arranged counterclockwise around the main deity—Citrasenā, Kāminī, Pātālavāsinī and Saubhadrā—correspond to Akṣobhya, Vairocana, Ratnasambhava and Amitābha respectively.

33. Six-deity Mahāmāyā-maṇḍala

Pattern: 16. Eight-petalled lotus;
Colour scheme:
Yoga tantras
centred on Vairocana

AMM: No. 58; VA: No. 9

The *Mahāmāyā-tantra* is one of the Mother tantras of the Highest Yoga tantras, and Heruka, the main deity of this tantra, is usually called Mahāmāyā. The *Abhisamayamuktāmālā* describes three kinds of Mahāmāyā-maṇḍala, large, medium and small, and this maṇḍala corresponds to the large version, while the other two are included in the *Mitra brgya rtsa* handscroll (M-60, 61). This maṇḍala takes the form of a red eight-petalled lotus, on the pericarp of which four-headed and four-armed Mahāmāyā accompanied by his consort Buddhaḍākinī is depicted as the main deity. On the lotus petals in the four cardinal directions are the four *ḍākinī*s Vajraḍākinī (east), Ratnaḍākinī (south), Padmaḍākinī (west) and Viśvaḍākinī (north). The Hahn Foundation handscroll depicts small circles representing the seats for deities in the intermediate directions too. However, these circles are not the seats for deities, but vases and *kapāla*s depicted on the lotus petals in the intermediate directions. lCaṅ skya II gives the number of deities as five, whereas the *Abhisamayamuktāmālā* includes the consort of the main deity, making a total of six. Mahāmāyā belongs to the Vajra family presided over by Akṣobhya, but his consort Buddhaḍākinī belongs to the Buddha family presided over by Vairocana, and the four *ḍākinī*s in the four cardinal directions belong to the Vajra, Jewel, Lotus and Action families respectively. Therefore, the colour scheme of the courtyard is the same as that of the Yoga tantras centred on Vairocana (Type A).

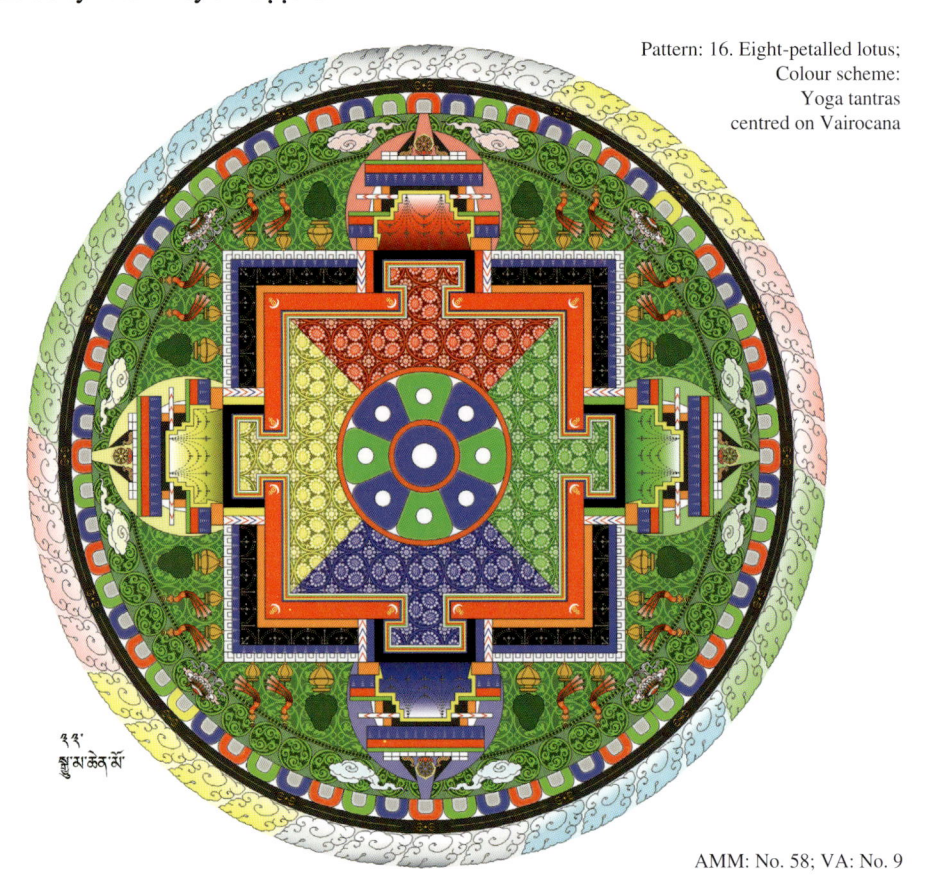

34. Fifty-eight-deity Yogāmbara-maṇḍala

Pattern: 23. Nine-panel grid;
Colour scheme:
Highest Yoga tantras
centred on Akṣobhya

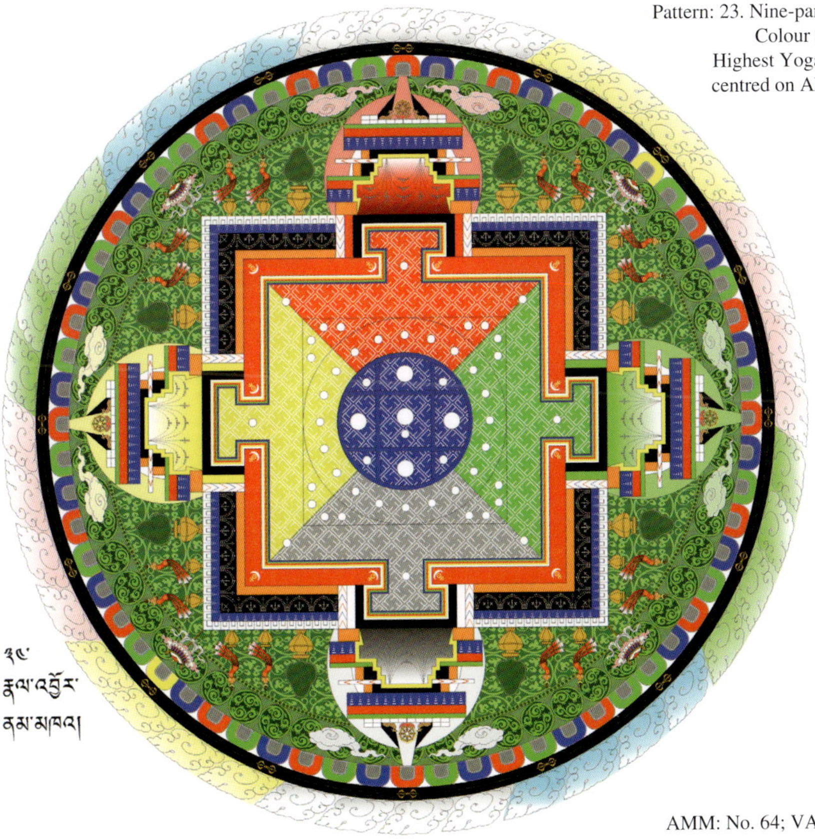

༣༩་
རྣལ་འབྱོར་
ནམ་མཁའ།

AMM: No. 64; VA: No. 14

This maṇḍala and the next one are both based on the *Catuṣpīṭha-tantra*, and it takes the form of a nine-panel grid, in the centre of which three-headed and six-armed Yogāmbara accompanied by his consort Jñānaḍākinī is depicted as the main deity. In the panels in the four cardinal directions are the four goddesses Vajraḍākinī (east), Ghoraḍākinī (north), Vetālī (west) and Caṇḍālī (south), and in the four intermediate directions are the four animal-headed goddesses Siṃhinī (Lion-headed, northeast), Vyāghrī (Tiger-headed, southeast), Jambukī (Wild-dog-headed, southwest) and Ulūkī (Owl-headed, northwest). Behind the four goddesses in the cardinal directions are the four goddesses Ḍākinī (east), Dīpinī (north), Cūṣinī (west) and Kāmbojī (south), although their seats are missing in the Hahn Foundation handscroll. In the outer circle are twenty goddesses, starting with Pukkasī, and outside the circle are twenty-four Hindu gods, starting with Hari (Viṣṇu). Thus, the total number of deities is fifty-seven. The *Patraratnamālā* gives the number of deities as fifty-seven, whereas lCaṅ skya II includes the consort of the main deity, making a total of fifty-eight. The colour scheme of the courtyard is that of the Highest Yoga tantras centred on Akṣobhya (Type E).

35. Thirteen-deity Jñānaḍākinī-maṇḍala

Pattern: 24. Nine-panel grid;
Colour scheme:
special type

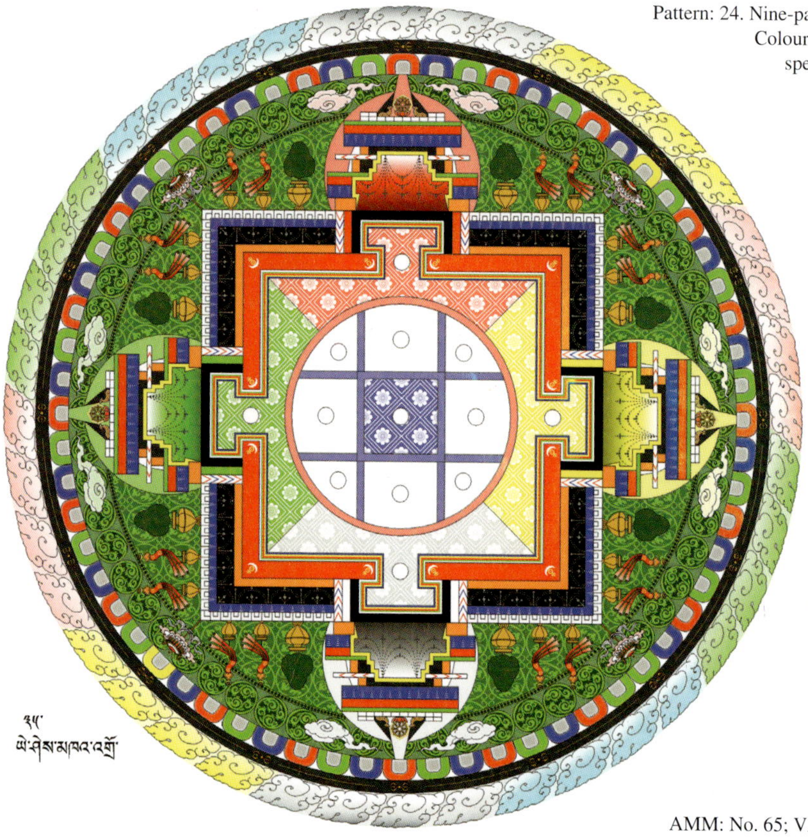

AMM: No. 65; VA: No. 4

The Jñānaḍākinī-maṇḍala, based on the *Catuṣpīṭha-tantra*, takes the form of a nine-panel grid, in the centre of which three-headed and six-armed Jñānaḍākinī is depicted as the main deity. In the panels in the four cardinal directions the four goddesses Vajraḍākinī (east), Ghoraḍākinī (north), Vetālī (west) and Caṇḍālī (south) are arranged counterclockwise, and in the four intermediate directions are the four animal-headed goddesses Siṃhinī (northeast), Vyāghrī (southeast), Jambukī (southwest) and Ulūkī (northwest), while the four gates are occupied by the four female gatekeepers Rājendrī (east), Dīpinī (north), Cūṣinī (west) and Kāmbojī (south). Thus, this maṇḍala consists of thirteen deities. The Hahn Foundation handscroll adopts an unusual colour scheme for the courtyard consisting of white (east), green (south), red (west) and yellow (north). This colour scheme is a mirror image of that of the Highest Yoga tantras centred on Akṣobhya. This is because the four goddesses arranged around the main deity—Vajraḍākinī, Ghoraḍākinī, Vetālī and Caṇḍālī, who correspond to Vairocana, Ratnasambhava, Amitābha and Amoghasiddhi respectively—are arranged not clockwise, as is normal, but counterclockwise.

36. Kāyavākcittaparinispanna-Kālacakra-mandala

Pattern: Composite type;
Colour scheme:
Kālacakra

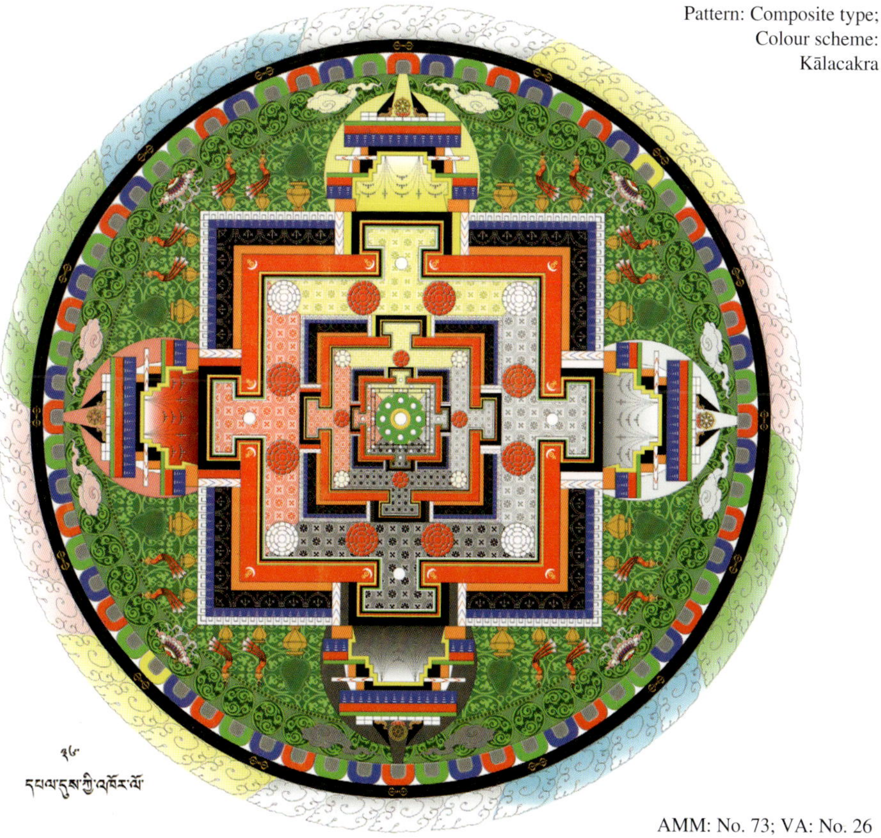

༣༦་
དཔལ་དུས་ཀྱི་འཁོར་ལོ་

AMM: No. 73; VA: No. 26

The *Kālacakra-tantra* belongs to the last phase of Tantric Buddhism. In Tibet, it is styled a "nondual tantra," synthesizing the theories of the earlier Father and Mother tantras. Among the many maṇḍalas of India and Tibet, the Kayavākcittaparinispanna-Kalacakra-maṇḍala, described in Chapter 3 of the *Kālacakra-tantra*, is the largest, and it could be said to represent the culmination of the historical development of the maṇḍala. This maṇḍala has a threefold structure, symbolizing body, speech and mind. On the pericarp of the eight-petalled lotus in the centre of the mind-maṇḍala, Kālacakra accompanied by his consort Viśvamātā is depicted as the main deity. On the eight lotus petals surrounding the main deity are eight goddesses, starting with Kṛṣṇadīptā, and outside the lotus four Buddhas, four Buddha-mothers, six bodhisattvas, six adamantine goddesses and six wrathful deities (two of them placed outside the pavilion), the basic constituent members of this maṇḍala, are depicted. The iconometry and design of the square pavilions differ greatly from those of other maṇḍalas, but in the Hahn Foundation handscroll they are depicted in the standard manner. This maṇḍala adopts a most unusual colour scheme for the courtyard, consisting of black (east), red (south), yellow (west) and white (north) (Type D). This colour scheme is based on the unique system of the *Kālacakra-tantra*, which unifies cosmology and maṇḍala theory.

37. Fifty-three-deity Vajradhātu-maṇḍala

Pattern: 25. Four-petalled lotus + nine-panel grid;
Colour scheme:
Yoga tantras
centred on Vairocana

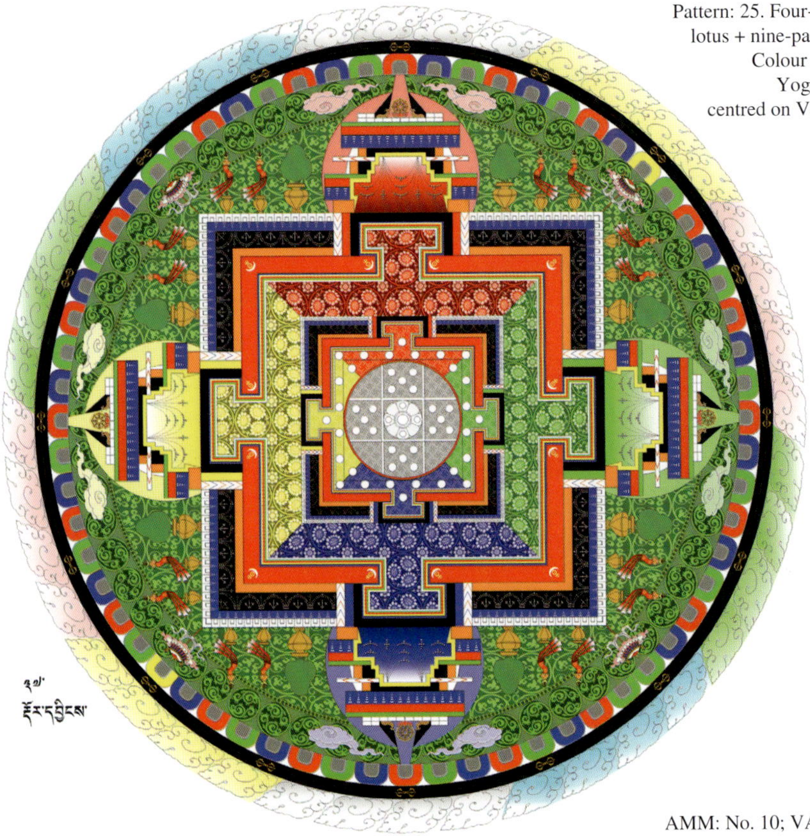

༣༧་
རྡོར་དབྱིངས་

AMM: No. 10; VA: No. 19

The Vajradhātu-maṇḍala, one of the Sino-Japanese Two World maṇḍalas, is regarded as the basic maṇḍala of the Yoga tantras. According to *Roṅ tha's Iconometry*, it takes the form of a four-petalled lotus arranged in a nine-panel grid. Vajradhātu-Vairocana is depicted in the centre, and on the lotus petals in the four cardinal directions the four *pāramitā*s Sattvavajrī (east), Ratnavajrī (south), Dharmavajrī (west) and Karmavajrī (north) are arranged around the main deity. On the panels in the four cardinal directions are the four Buddhas and sixteen great bodhisattvas: Akṣobhya, Vajrasattva, Vajrarāja, Vajrarāga and Vajrasādhu (east), Ratnasambhava, Vajraratna, Vajrateja, Vajraketu and Vajrahāsa (south), Amitābha, Vajradharma, Vajratīkṣṇa, Vajrahetu and Vajrabhāṣa (west), and Amoghasiddhi, Vajrakarma, Vajrarakṣa, Vajrayakṣa and Vajrasandhi (north). In the four intermediate directions are the four inner offering goddesses Vajralāsyā, Vajramālā, Vajragītā and Vajranṛtyā and the four outer offering goddesses Vajradhūpā, Vajrapuṣpā, Vajradīpā and Vajragandhā. In the surrounding strips of the inner pavilion, the sixteen bodhisattvas of the Auspicious Aeon (Bhadrakalpa) are arranged, and in the four gates of the inner maṇḍala are the four gatekeepers Vajrāṅkuśa, Vajrapāśa, Vajrasphoṭa and Vajrāveśa. Thus, this maṇḍala consists of fifty-three deities. However, in the Hahn Foundation handscroll a blank space has been left inside the outer pavilion, and this seems to be for the Thousand Buddhas of the Auspicious Aeon. While the colour scheme of the courtyard ought to be that of the Yoga tantras centred on Vairocana (Type A), in the Hahn Foundation handscroll the colours of south and north have been wrongly changed, but here they have been corrected with reference to other examples of this maṇḍala.

38. Thirty-seven-deity Navoṣṇīṣa-maṇḍala

Pattern: 28a. Eight petalled lotus + eight-spoked wheel; Colour scheme: special type

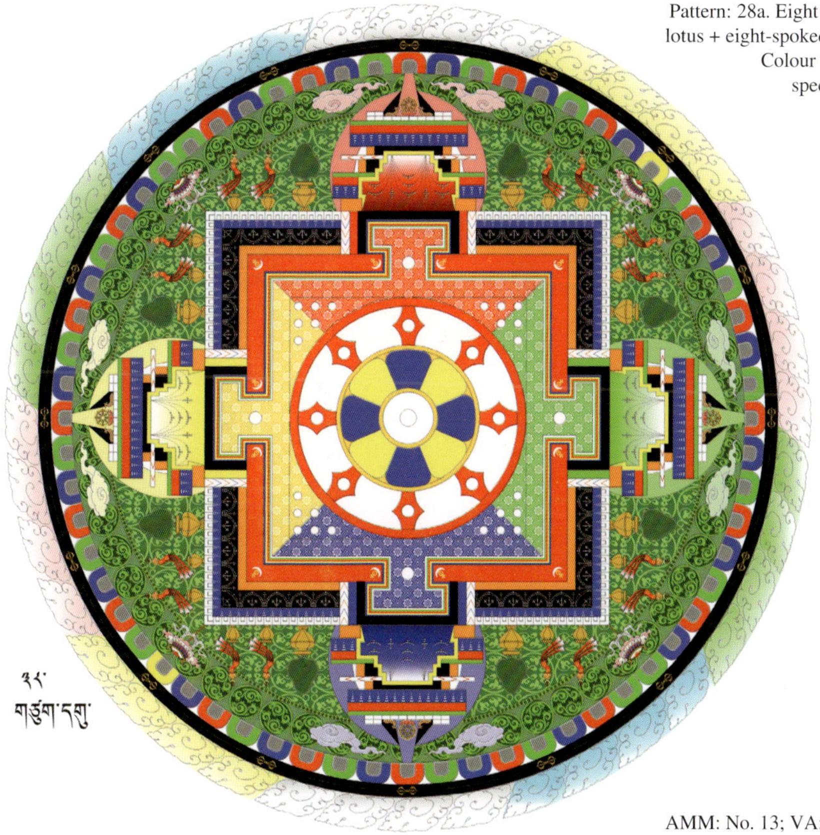

AMM: No. 13; VA: No. 22

The Navoṣṇīṣa-maṇḍala is the first and one of the basic maṇḍalas explained in the new translation of the *Sarvadurgatipariśodhana-tantra*. It takes the form of an eight-petalled lotus set on the hub of an eight-spoked wheel. Śākyamuni is depicted in the centre of the eight-petalled lotus, and the eight *uṣṇīṣa* deities Vajroṣṇīṣa (east), Ratnoṣṇīṣa (south), Padmoṣṇīṣa (west), Viśvoṣṇīṣa (north), Tejoṣṇīṣa (southeast), Dhvajoṣṇīṣa (southwest), Tīkṣṇoṣṇīṣa (northwest) and Chatroṣṇīṣa (northeast) are arranged on the eight spokes of the wheel. In the four intermediate directions are the eight offering goddesses, in the four gates are four gatekeepers, and in the surrounding strips of the pavilion are the sixteen bodhisattvas of the Auspicious Aeon (Bhadrakalpa). Thus, the total number of deities is thirty-seven. Examples of this maṇḍala are common in Tibet, but most of them lack the eight-petalled lotus on the hub of the wheel. However, early examples from Alci and Dung dkar Cave No. 3 show an eight-petalled lotus in the centre. This would suggest that the Hahn Foundation handscroll and *Roṅ tha's Iconometry* preserve an old tradition. The Hahn Foundation handscroll adopts an unusual colour scheme for the courtyard consisting of blue (east), white (south), red (west) and green (north). But this would seem to be an error since no textual source has been found for it, and it has therefore been changed to accord with the colour scheme of the Yoga tantras centred on Vairocana. However, there exists another colour scheme—white (east), blue (south), red (west) and green (north)—to coincide with the body colours of the four *uṣṇīṣa* deities.

39. Dharmadhātuvāgīśvara-maṇḍala

Pattern: 26. Nine-panel grid;
Colour scheme:
Yoga tantras
centred on Vairocana

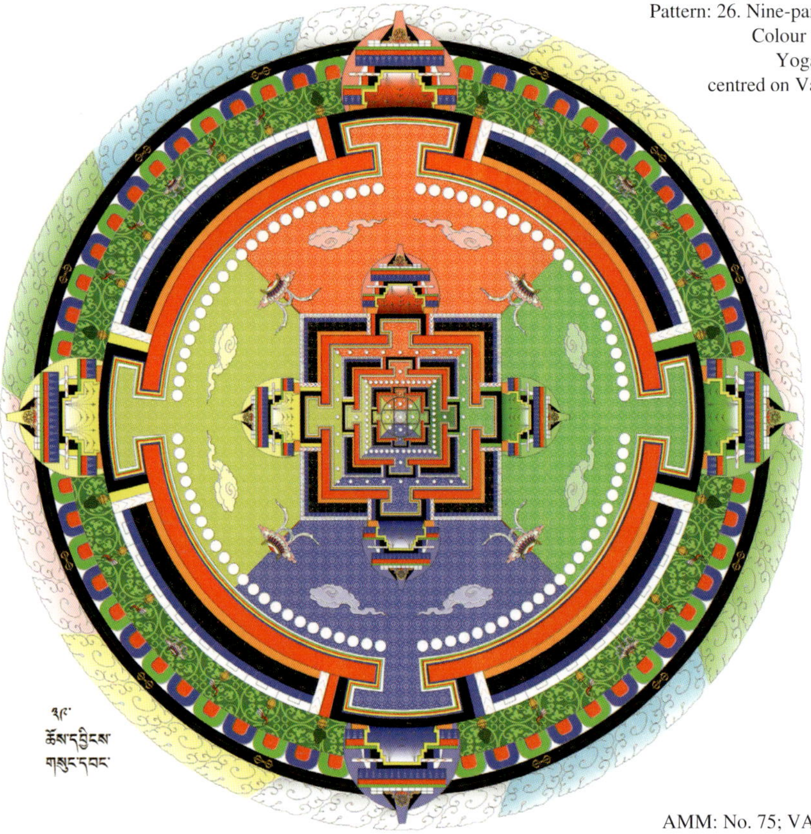

༣༨་
ཆོས་དབྱིངས་
གསུང་དབང་

AMM: No. 75; VA: No. 21

The Dharmadhātuvāgīśvara-maṇḍala is a large-scale maṇḍala based on the *Mañjuśrīnāmasaṅgīti*. It has a quadruple structure, and in the centre of the eight-petalled lotus in the central panel of the nine-panel grid in the innermost pavilion four-headed and eight-armed Dharmadhātuvāgīśvara-Mañjuśrī is depicted as the main deity. On the lotus petals surrounding the main deity are the eight *uṣṇīṣa* deities. In the panels in the four cardinal directions are the four Buddhas Akṣobhya, Ratnasambhava, Amitābha and Amoghasiddhi, each attended by four of the sixteen great bodhisattvas; in the panels in the intermediate directions are the four Buddha-mothers Locanā, Māmakī, Pāṇḍarā and Tārā; and in the four gates are the four gatekeepers starting with Vajrāṅkuśa. In the second pavilion are deifications of doctrinal categories of Buddhism: twelve *bhūmi*s (east), twelve *pāramitā*s (south), twelve *vaśitā*s (west), twelve *dhāraṇī*s (north) and four *pratisaṃvit*s (in the four gates). In the four intermediate directions are the four inner offering goddesses, while the sixteen bodhisattvas of the Auspicious Aeon (Bhadrakalpa) and eight wrathful deities are arranged in the third pavilion, and many protective deities are arranged around the outermost circle. Thus, the total number of deities is either 119 or 220. This maṇḍala could be said to represent the culmination of the historical development of the maṇḍalas of the Yoga tantras. In the Hahn Foundation handscroll this maṇḍala alone occupies two registers rather than one so as to show all its details. The colour scheme of the courtyard is that of the Yoga tantras centred on Vairocana (Type A).

40. Thirty-four-deity Bhūtaḍāmara-maṇḍala

Pattern: 37. Nine-panel grid;
Colour scheme:
Highest Yoga tantras
centred on Akṣobhya

༤༠་
འབྱུང་པོ་འདུལ་
བྱེད་

AMM: not described; VA: No. 23

Among the maṇḍalas described in the *Vajrāvalī*, this is the only maṇḍala that is classified among the Caryā tantras, although it is not related to the *Vairocanābhisambodhi-sūtra*, the root scripture of the Caryā tantras. According to *Roṅ tha's Iconometry*, this maṇḍala takes the form of a nine-panel grid surrounded by a double square. In the centre, four-armed Bhūtaḍāmara is depicted as the main deity. In the eight directions surrounding the main deity are eight Hindu deities: Maheśvara (east), Viṣṇu (south), Brahmā (west), Kārttikeya (north), Gaṇapati (northeast), Ravi (southeast), Rāhu (southwest) and Nandikeśvara (northwest). In the second square are the Hindu goddesses Śrī (east), Tilottamā (south), Śaśī (west), Umā (north), Ratnaśrī (southeast), Sarasvatī (southwest), Surasundarī (northwest) and Ābhūtī (northeast); in the third square are the protectors of the directions, starting with Indra (in the northeast, Īśāna is accompanied by Candra); and in the outermost square are eight goddesses, starting with Siṃhadhvajadhāriṇī. The colour scheme of the courtyard is that of the Highest Yoga tantras centred on Akṣobhya (Type E) since Bhūtaḍāmara is an emanation of Vajrapāṇi, who belongs to the Vajra family.

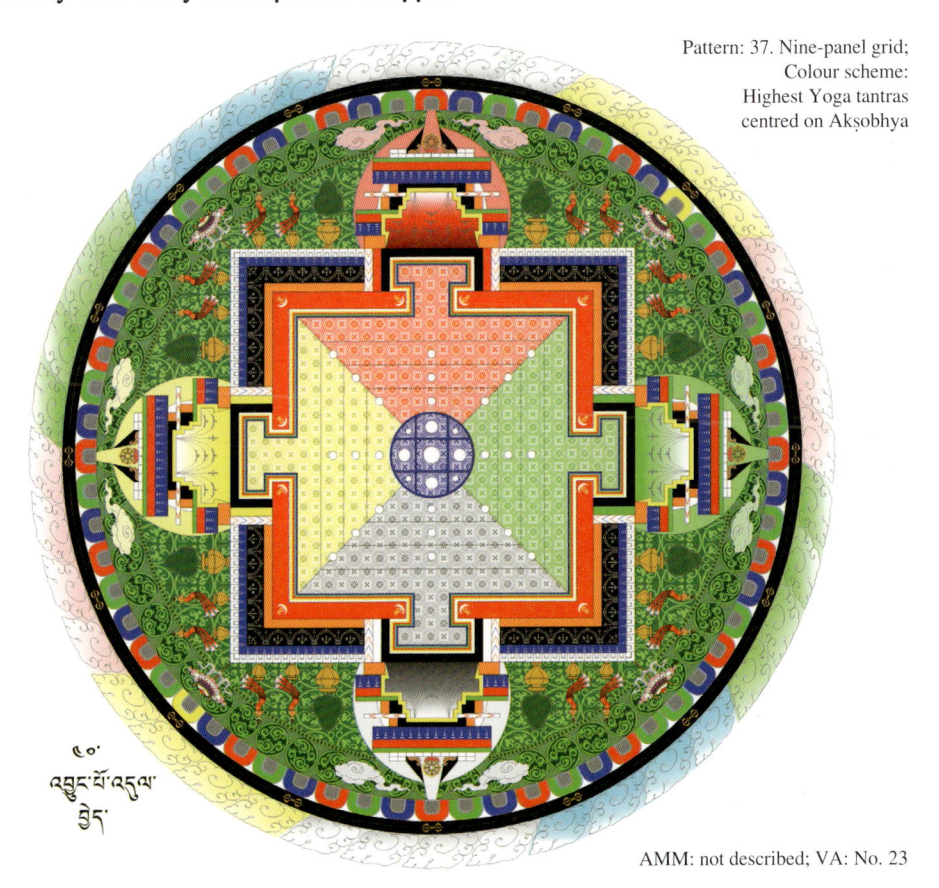

41. Twenty-five-deity Mārīcī-maṇḍala

Pattern: 41a. Eight-petalled lotus;
Colour scheme:
Yoga tantras
centred on Vairocana

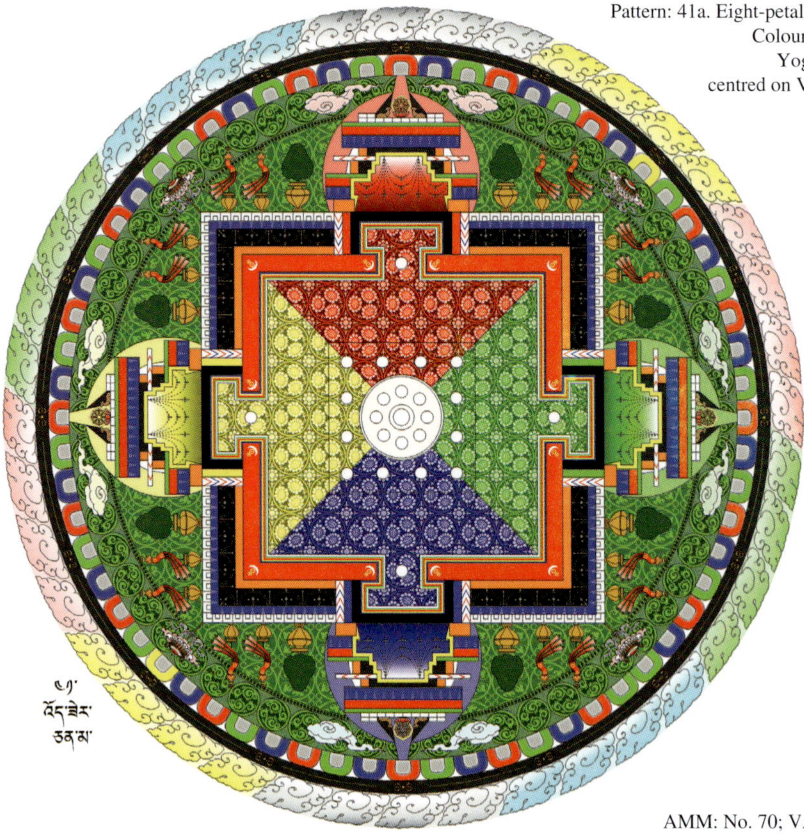

༤༡་
འོད་ཟེར་
ཅན་མ་

AMM: No. 70; VA: No. 17

Mārīcī is a goddess personifying the mirage. She was widely worshipped for the purpose of averting attacks from enemies and thieves since, it is said, no one, not even the sun, can see her even though she always goes before the sun. According to *Roṅ tha's Iconometry*, this maṇḍala takes the form of an eight-petalled lotus, on the pericarp of which three-headed and six-armed Mārīcī is depicted. On the lotus petals in the eight directions are Arkamasi (east), Markamasi (south), Antardhānamasi (west), Tejomasi (north), Udayamasi (southeast), Gulmamasi (southwest), Vanamasi (northwest) and Cīvaramasi (northeast). In the outer circle are the eight goddesses Mahācīvaramasi, Varāhamukhī (east), Padākramasi, Varale (south), Parākramasi, Vadale (west), Ūrmamasi and Varāli (north), in the four intermediate directions are the four goddesses Vatāli (southeast), Vadāli (southwest), Varāli (northwest) and Varāhamukhi (northeast), and in the four gates are the four female gatekeepers Ālo (east), Tālo (south), Kālo (west) and Satsalosambamūrdhaṭī (north). Their unusual names are deifications of phrases occurring in Mārīcī's *dhāraṇī*.

42. Thirteen-deity Pañcarakṣā-maṇḍala

Pattern: 42.
Nine four-petalled lotuses;
Colour scheme:
special type

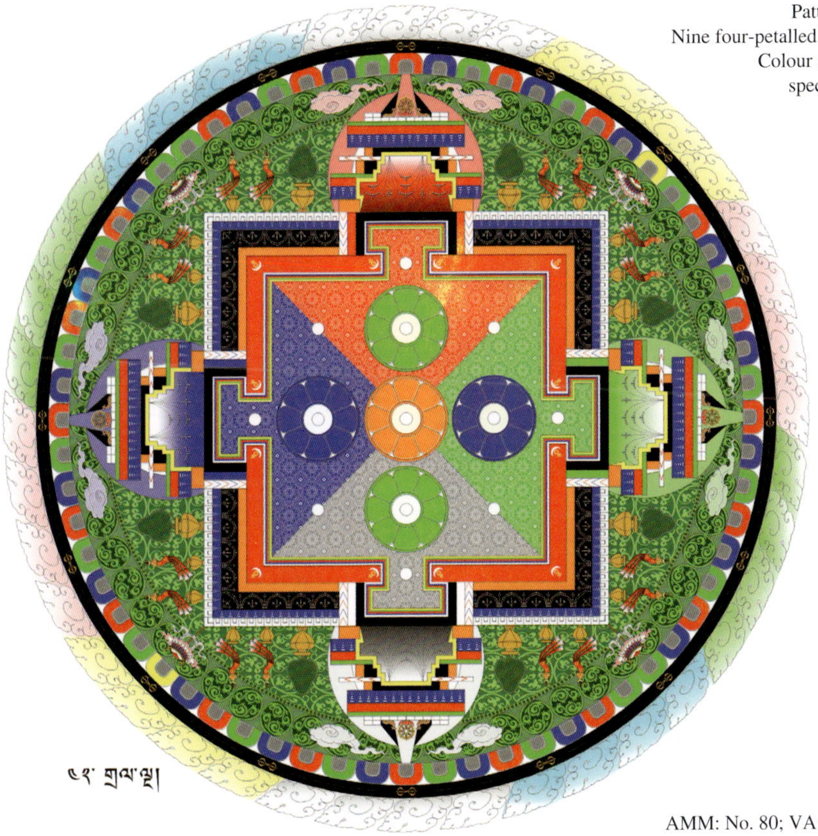

༤༢་ གྲལ་ལྷ།

AMM: No. 80; VA: No. 18

The Pañcarakṣā, or "Five Protectresses," represent deifications of five well-known *dhāraṇīs* belonging to the Kriyā tantras, and they were widely worshipped in India and Tibet. This maṇḍala takes the form of eight-petalled lotuses arranged in the centre and in the four cardinal directions. On the lotus in the centre Mahāpratisarā is depicted as the main deity, and on the lotuses in the four cardinal directions are Mahāsahasrapramardanī (east), Mahāmantrānusāriṇī (south), Mahāśītavatī (west) and Mahāmāyūrī (north). In the four corners of the courtyard are Kālī (southeast), Kālarātrī (southwest), Kālakarṇī (northwest) and Śvetā (northeast), and in the four gates are the four female gatekeepers Aṅkuśī, Pāśī, Sphoṭā and Ghaṇṭā. Thus, this maṇḍala consists of thirteen deities. The *Abhisamayamuktāmālā*, on the other hand, describes a seventeen-deity maṇḍala, different from this maṇḍala, while *Roṅ tha's Iconometry* prescribes nine four-petalled lotuses in the courtyard. Thus, it is evident that there were several different renderings of this maṇḍala. The colour scheme of the courtyard is that of the Highest Yoga tantras centred on Ratnasambhava (Type G) since, according to the *Niṣpannayogāvalī*, Mahāpratisarā corresponds to Ratneśa (Ratnasambhava) and the four other goddesses starting with Mahāsahasrapramardanī correspond to Vairocana, etc.

43. Nineteen-deity Vasudhārā-maṇḍala

Pattern: 46. Eight-petalled lotus;
Colour scheme:
Highest Yoga tantras
centred on Ratnasambhava

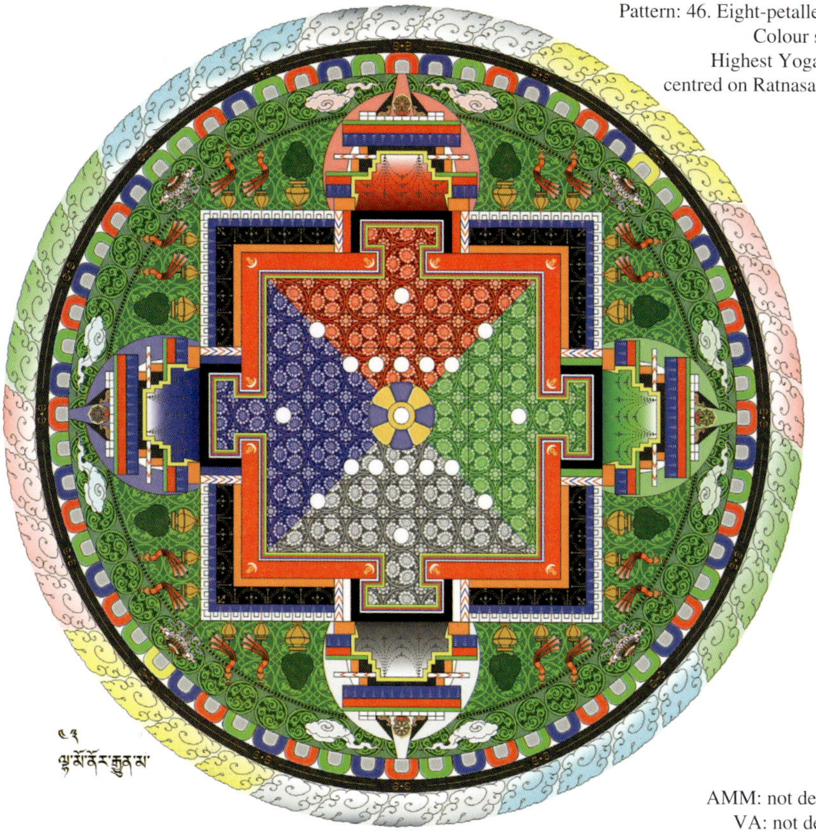

༤༣
ལྷ་མོ་ནོར་རྒྱུན་མ་

AMM: not described;
VA: not described

The following three maṇḍalas are explained neither in the *Vajrāvalī* nor in the *Abhisamayamuktāmālā* and have been supplemented from another ritual manual, the *Kriyāsamuccaya*. In these three maṇḍalas, there are considerable differences in design with extant examples of the *Vajrāvalī* set, and therefore these versions have been created mainly with reference to the Hahn Foundation handscroll. Vasudhārā is the consort of Jambhala, a god of wealth, and in India and Tibet she is widely worshipped as a goddess of fertility. This maṇḍala takes the form of an eight-petalled lotus surrounded by a double square, with the main deity Vasudhārā depicted on the pericarp of the lotus. In the east and west of the second square are six deities, starting with Vajradharasāgaranirghoṣa, and in the four intermediate directions four *yakṣa*s, starting with Civikuṇḍalin. In the four intermediate directions of the third square are four goddesses, starting with Guptadevī, and four *yakṣa*s, starting with Pūrṇabhadra. Thus, this maṇḍala consists of nineteen deities. The Hahn Foundation handscroll shows a four-petalled lotus in the centre, but this has been changed to an eight-petalled lotus by referring to *Roṅ tha's Iconometry* and other examples of the *Vajrāvalī* set. The colour scheme of the courtyard is that of the Highest Yoga tantras centred on Ratnsambhava (Type G) since Vasudhārā belongs to the Jewel family presided over by Ratnasambhava.

44. Twenty-one-deity Grahamātṛkā-maṇḍala

Pattern: 49b. Eight-petalled lotus;
Colour scheme:
Yoga tantras
centred on Vairocana

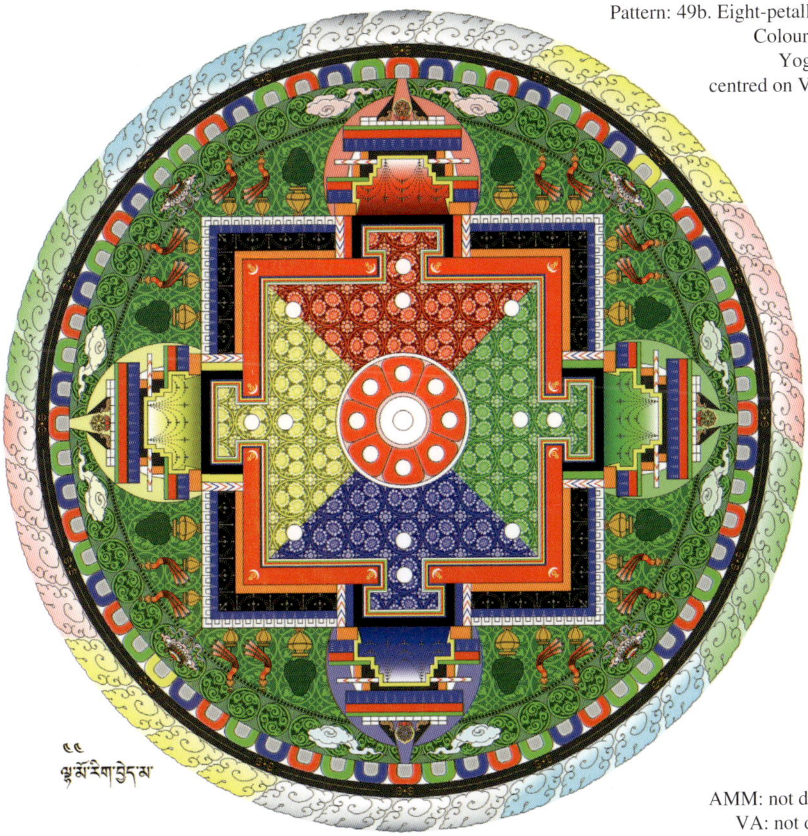

༤༤
ལྷ་མོ་རིག་བྱེད་མ་

AMM: not described;
VA: not described

Among the three maṇḍalas supplemented from the *Kriyāsamuccaya*, this maṇḍala exhibits the largest differences in design, and this version has been created mainly with reference to the Hahn Foundation handscroll. This maṇḍala is based on the cult of planets. However, the main deity is not the Sun depicted in the centre, but a goddess named Grahamātṛkā or Mahāvidyā (Great Knowledge) in the northwest corner. This maṇḍala takes the form of an eight-petalled lotus, with the Sun on its pericarp. On the eight petals of the lotus are eight planets: Moon (east), Mars (south), Mercury (west), Jupiter (north), Venus (southeast), Saturn (southwest), Rāhu (northwest) and Ketu (northeast). In the four cardinal directions of the outer square are Buddha (east), Vajrapāṇi (south), Lokeśvara (west) and Mañjuśrī (north); in the four corners of the courtyard are all planets (northeast), all constellations (southeast), all disasters (southwest) and Grahamātṛkā, the main deity of this maṇḍala; and in the four gates are the four celestial kings Dhṛtarāṣṭra, Virūḍhaka, Virūpākṣa and Vaiśravaṇa. Thus, this maṇḍala consists of twenty-one deities. Other examples of this maṇḍala sometimes depict all the planets, constellations and disasters individually, but in the Hahn Foundation handscroll they are each represented by a single deity. The colour scheme of the courtyard is that of the Yoga tantras centred on Vairocana (Type A).

45. Thirty-three-deity Uṣṇīṣavijayā-maṇḍala

Pattern: 44b. Four-petalled lotus + eight-spoked wheel;
Colour scheme: Yoga tantras centred on Vairocana

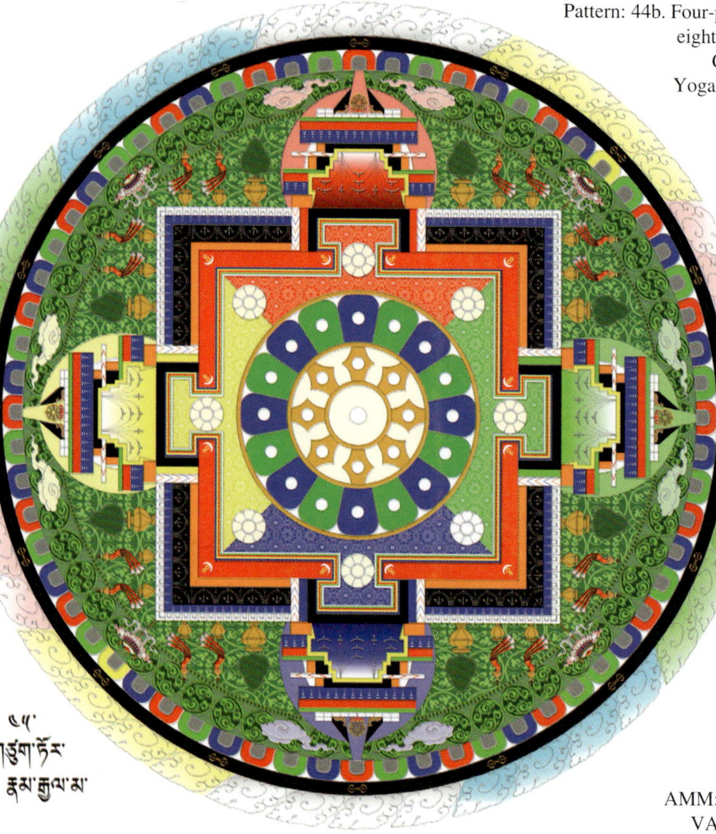

༤༥་
གཙུག་ཏོར་
རྣམ་རྒྱལ་མ་

AMM: not described;
VA: not described

The goddess Uṣṇīṣavijayā is a deification of the *Uṣṇīṣavijayā-dhāraṇī*, and she is counted as one of the "Three Deities of Longevity" together with Aparimitāyus and White Tārā. The handscroll of the *Mitra brgya rtsa* includes a nine-deity Uṣṇīṣavijayā-maṇḍala (M-4). The present maṇḍala, on the other hand, consists of thirty-three deities and takes the form of a sixteen-petalled lotus arranged around an eight-spoked wheel, on the hub of which Uṣṇīṣavijayā is depicted as the main deity. On the eight spokes are eight *uṣṇīṣa* deities, starting with Gaganasannibhodayoṣṇīṣa. These eight *uṣṇīṣa* deities seem to correspond to the four Buddhas and four Buddha-mothers of the Guhyasamāja-maṇḍala. On the sixteen petals of the lotus are *uṣṇīṣa* deities representing deifications of the sixteen types of *śūnyatā* expounded in the *Prajñāpāramitā-sūtra*. In the four corners of the courtyard and in the four gates are small eight-petalled lotuses. On four lotuses in the cardinal directions are four forms of Uṣṇīṣavijayā who conquer the four demons of obstacles (east), death (south), afflictions (west) and aggregates (north), and in the intermediate directions are four goddesses, starting with Vajramālāyurdātrī. The colour scheme of the courtyard is that of the Yoga tantras centred on Vairocana (Type A). The main deities of these three maṇḍalas supplemented from the *Kriyāsamuccaya*, Grahamātṛkā, Vasudhārā and Uṣṇīṣavijayā, are the main deities of the *burha-junko*, or celebration of longevity, which is held three times during the lifetime of Nepalese Buddhists. This would suggest that the *Kriyāsamuccaya* was compiled in Nepal.

Explanatory Remarks on
the *Mitra brgya rtsa* Set of Maṇḍalas

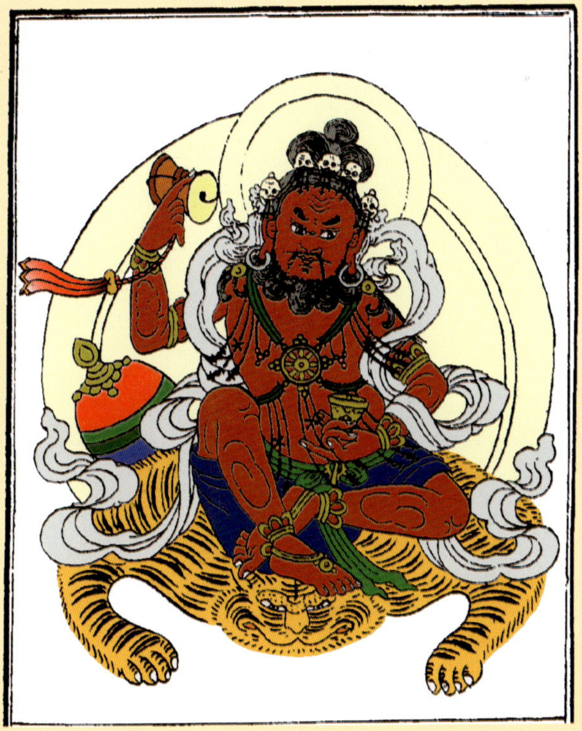

Mitrayogin

1. Thirteen-deity Sarasvatī-maṇḍala

Pattern: 45. Four-spoked wheel;
Colour scheme:
Yoga tantras
centred on Vairocana

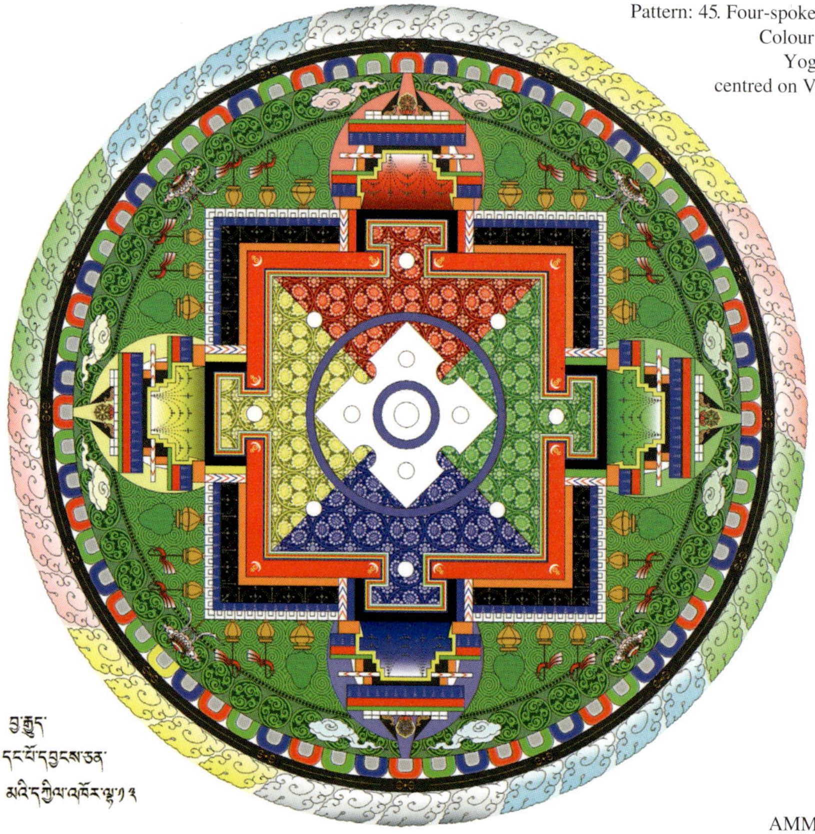

བྱ་རྒྱུད་
དང་པོ་དབྱངས་ཅན་
མའི་དཀྱིལ་འཁོར་ལྷ་༡༣

AMM: No. 71

In Tibet, Sarasvatī is revered as a goddess of learning and art. This maṇḍala takes the form of a four-spoked wheel, on the hub of which Sarasvatī is depicted as the main deity. On the spokes in the four cardinal directions are the four *pāramitā* goddesses Sattvavajrī (east), Ratnavajrī (south), Dharmavajrī (west) and Karmavajrī (north). In the four corners are the four inner offering goddesses Lāsyā, Mālā, Gītā and Nṛtyā, and in the four gates are the four female gatekeepers Aṅkuśī, Pāśī, Sphoṭā and Ghanṭā. Thus, this maṇḍala consists of thirteen deities, and Sarasvatī is accompanied by the same attendant deities as those in the Vajradhātu-maṇḍala. This suggests that Sarasvatī, originally a protective deity, was highly revered in Tibet and was chosen as the tutelary deity of learning for eminent monks. That all the attendants are female is possibly because Sarasvatī, the main deity, is a goddess. As in the Vajradhātu-maṇḍala (V-37), the colour scheme of the courtyard is that of the Yoga tantras centred on Vairocana (Type A). Examples of this maṇḍala are not common in Tibet, but in Japan rGyud smad Tantric College, exiled in India, has created a three-dimensional maṇḍala of Sarasvatī for Benten-shū, a new Buddhist sect centred on Sarasvatī.

2. Five-deity Parṇaśavarī-maṇḍala

Pattern: 48. Four-spoked wheel;
Colour scheme:
Highest Yoga tantras
centred on Akṣobhya

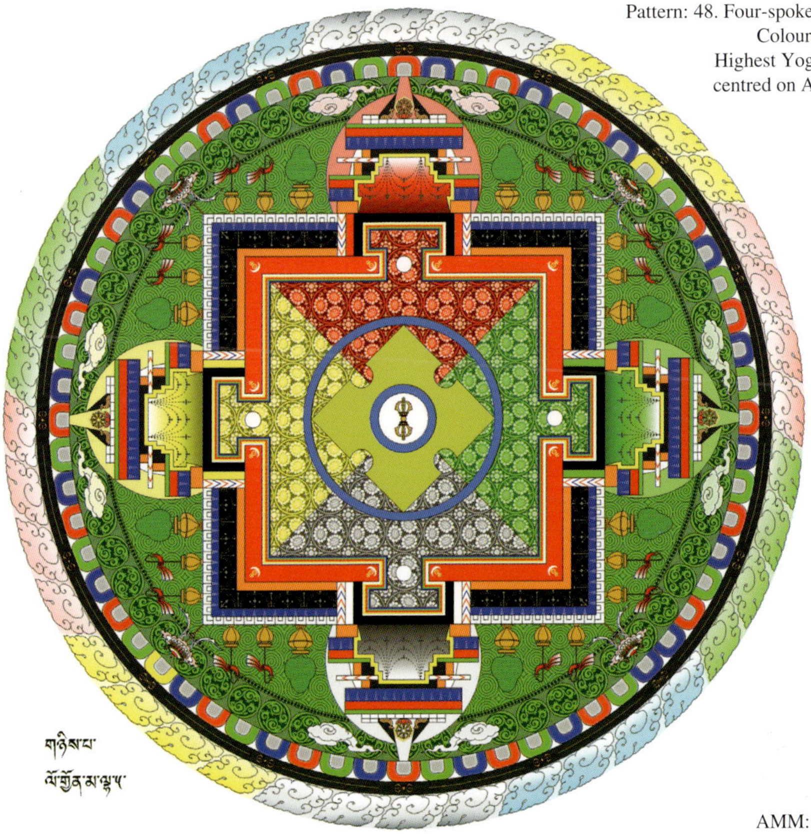

གཉིས་པ་
ལོ་གྱོན་མ་ལྔ་པ་

AMM: No. 106

The goddess Parṇaśavarī is a deification of the *Parṇaśavarī-dhāraṇī*. The *Sādhanamālā* describes her as either three-headed and four-armed or three-headed and six-armed, and in Tibet there is also a three-headed and eight-armed form. In India, she was worshipped as a goddess who subdues outbreaks of epidemics, and several statues of her have been unearthed. In Japan, on the other hand, she was regarded as an emanation of Avalokiteśvara because she is depicted in the retinue of the Lotus family in the Garbhadhātu-maṇḍala, and she was also called Yōe Kannon (Leaf-clad Avalokiteśvara). In Japan, she is counted among thirty-three emanations of Avalokiteśvara, but she was not widely worshipped as an independent deity. According to *Roṅ tha's Iconometry*, her maṇḍala takes the form of a four-spoked wheel like the five-deity Amoghapāśa-maṇḍala (M-9), and three-headed and six-armed Parṇaśavarī (here represented by a vajra) is depicted on the hub as the main deity. In the four gates are the four celestial kings Dhṛtarāṣṭra (east), Virūḍhaka (south), Virūpākṣa (west) and Vaiśravaṇa (north). The colour scheme of the courtyard is that of the Highest Yoga tantras centred on Akṣobhya (Type E). The *Abhisamayamuktāmālā* explains that Parṇaśavarī belongs to the Vajra family presided over by Akṣobhya, and this colour scheme seems to accord with this. Examples of this maṇḍala are rare in Tibet.

3. Twenty-nine-deity Sitātapatrā-maṇḍala

Pattern: 43. Eight-petalled lotus + sixteen-spoked wheel;
Colour scheme:
Yoga tantras
centred on Vairocana

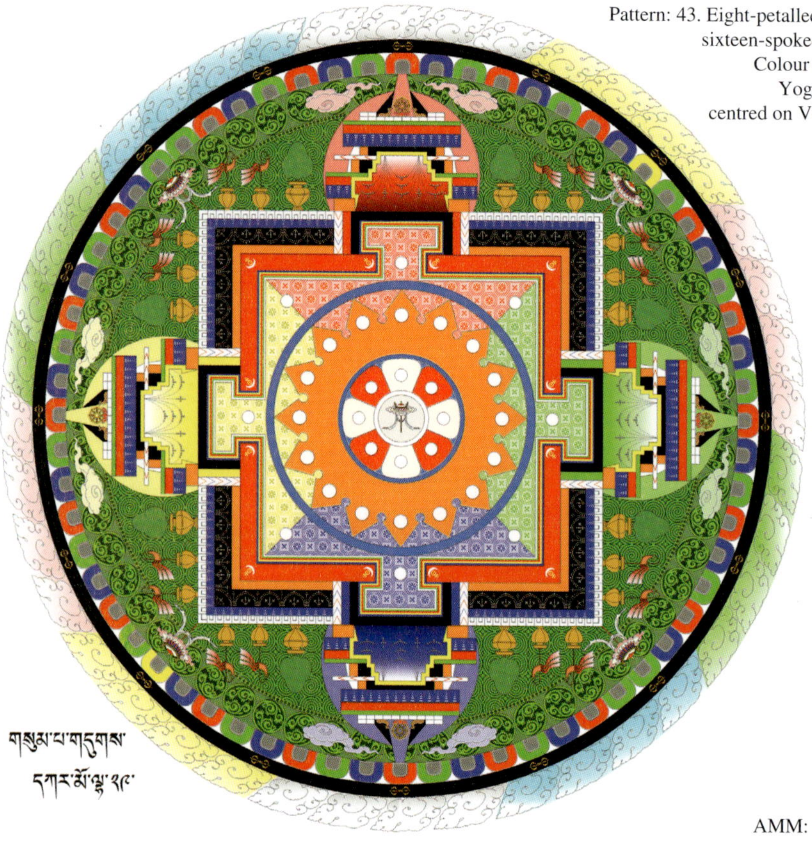

གསུམ་པ་གདུགས་
དཀར་མོ་ལྷ་༢༩་

AMM: No. 105

The goddess Sitātapatrā, or "White Parasol," is a deification of the *Sitātapatrā-dhāraṇī*, also known as the *Mahoṣṇīṣa-dhāraṇī* (Ch. *Lengyan zhou*). In Tibet, she is worshipped so as to protect the country from disasters. There are three forms of Sitātapatrā: one-headed and two-armed, three headed and six-armed or eight-armed, and thousand-headed and thousand-armed. These three forms are styled large, medium and small. The main deity of this maṇḍala assumes the three-headed and eight-armed form. This maṇḍala takes the form of an eight-petalled lotus surrounded by a sixteen-spoked wheel. On the pericarp of the eight-petalled lotus Sitātapatrā (here represented by a white parasol) is depicted as the main deity, while on the eight petals are Drag śul chen mo (east), gTum mo chen mo (south), 'Bar ma chen mo (west) and sTobs chen mo (north). On the sixteen spokes of the wheel are sixteen goddesses whose names are not widely known, but it turns out that they are emanations of Sitātapatrā explained in the *Sitātapatrā-dhāraṇī*. In the four gates are four wrathful gatekeepers identical to those in the thirty-three-deity Uṣṇīṣavijayā-maṇḍala (M-4). Thus, the total number of deities is twenty-nine. The colour scheme of the courtyard is that of the Yoga tantras centred on Vairocana (Type A) since Sitātapatrā belongs to the Tathāgata family presided over by Vairocana.

4. Nine-deity Uṣṇīṣavijayā-maṇḍala

Pattern: 44. Lotus + wheel;
Colour scheme:
Yoga tantras
centred on Vairocana

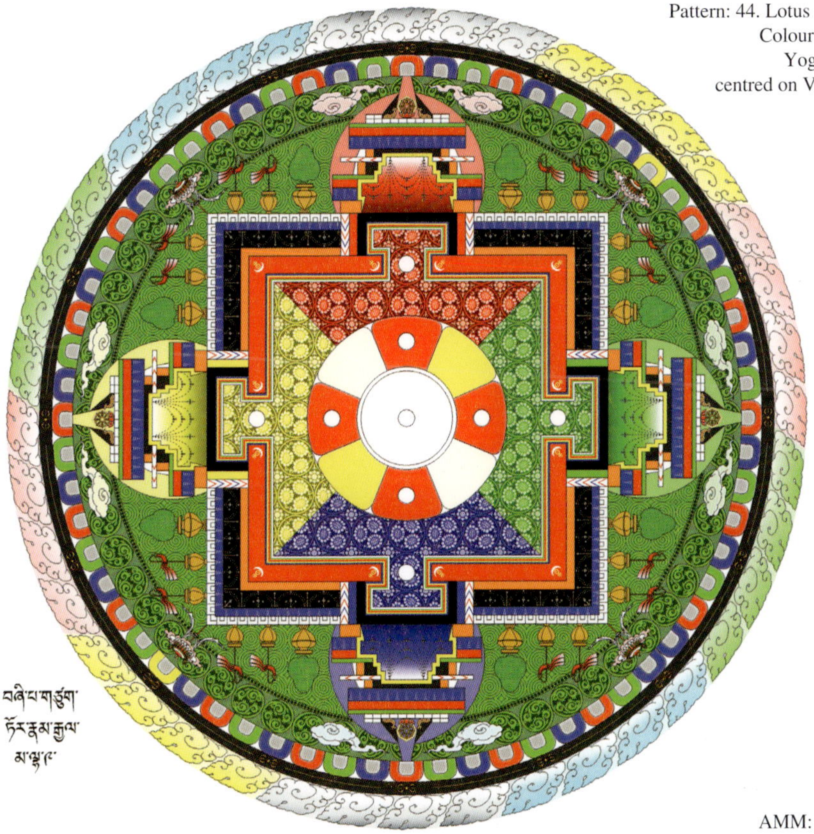

བཞི་པ་གཙུག་
ཏོར་རྣམ་རྒྱལ་
མ་ལྷ་༩་

AMM: No. 104

The goddess Uṣṇīṣavijayā is a deification of the *Uṣṇīṣavijayā-dhāraṇī*, and in Tibet she is worshipped as one of the Three Deities of Longevity (*Tshe lha rnam gsum*). This maṇḍala takes the form of an eight-petalled lotus, on the pericarp of which Uṣṇīṣavijayā is depicted as the main deity. On the four petals in the four cardinal directions are Avalokiteśvara (right), Vajrapāṇi-Guhyakādhipati (left) and two celestial beings. In the four gates are the four wrathful deities Acala, Ṭakkirāja, Nīladaṇḍa and Mahābala. The combination of Uṣṇīṣavijayā, Avalokiteśvara, Vajrapāṇi and four wrathful deities is explained in the *Sādhanamālā* (No. 211). Therefore, we can surmise that this maṇḍala represents a rearrangement of the deities of *Sādhanamālā* No. 211 so as to form a symmetrical maṇḍala, both horizontally and vertically, through the addition of two celestial beings. A similar combination of deities can also be seen in a relief in caves at Feilaifeng near Hangzhou, China, which started being excavated during the Zhiyuan era of the Yuan dynasty, and in clay figures in the rNam rgyal lha khang (Uṣṇīṣavijayā Chapel) on the first floor of the Great Stūpa of dPal 'khor chos sde in rGyal rtse. This present maṇḍala is important since it is a pictorial rendering of the deities of the Uṣṇīṣavijayā cycle rather than in sculpture. *Roṅ tha's Iconometry* explains the layout of this maṇḍala as a combination of a four-petalled lotus and an eight-spoked wheel, but this does not coincide with the Hahn Foundation handscroll.

5. Nine-deity Jambhala-maṇḍala

Pattern: 49a. Eight-petalled lotus;
Colour scheme:
Highest Yoga tantras
centred on
Ratnasambhava

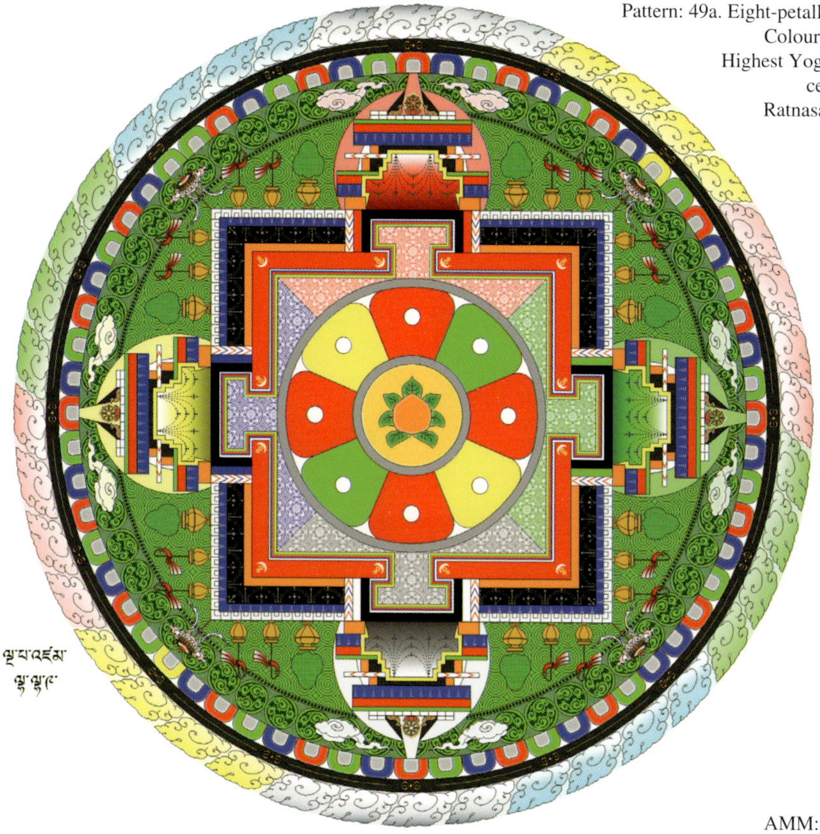

ལྷ་པ་འཛམ་
ལྷུ་ལྷུ་ཁ་

AMM: No. 107

Jambhala is a type of *yakṣa*, and in Tibet he is worshipped as a god of wealth. Generally speaking, the *yakṣa* has the twin aspects of a god of war and a god of wealth, and Jambhala is a deity in which his aspect as a god of wealth comes to the fore. His maṇḍala takes the form of an eight-petalled lotus. In the centre, Yellow Jambhala (here represented by a citron) is depicted together with his consort Vasudhārā. On the eight lotus petals are the eight *yakṣa* generals (*rta bdag brgyad*) Maṇibhadra, Pūrṇabhadra, Dhanada, Vaiśravaṇa, Caranendra/Carendraka, Kelimālin, Vicitrakuṇḍalin and Mukhendra. The colour scheme of the courtyard is that of the Highest Yoga tantras centred on Ratnasambhava (Type G) since Jambhala belongs to the Jewel family presided over by Ratnasambhava. No maṇḍala of Jambhala is included in the Ṅor maṇḍalas. However, a seed-syllable maṇḍala and a three-dimensional maṇḍala in which the eight *yakṣa* generals were arranged around Jambhala (with five *yakṣa* generals surviving) have been discovered in India. This suggests that Jambhala was widely worshipped as a god of wealth in India too.

6. Thirty-five-deity Śākyamuni-maṇḍala

Pattern: 40. Triple eight-petalled lotus;
Colour scheme:
Highest Yoga tantras
centred on
Ratnasambhava

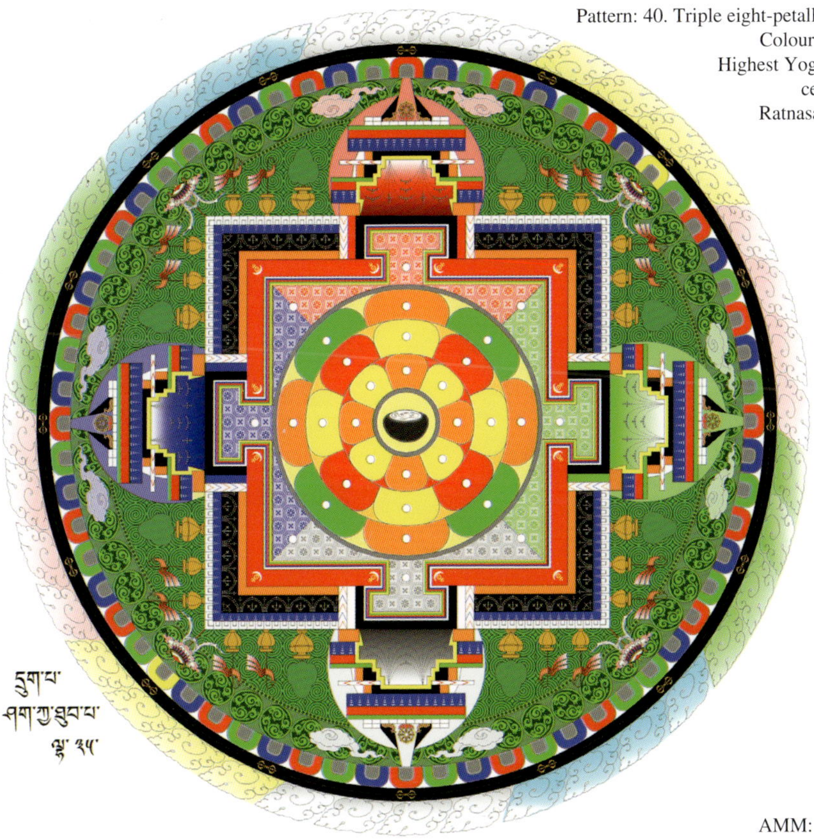

དྲུག་པ་
ཤག་ཀྱ་ཐུབ་པ་
ལྷ་ ༣༥་

AMM: No. 102

This is the only maṇḍala in the *Mitra brgya rtsa* set with Śākyamuni as the main deity. The *Abhisamayamuktāmālā* quotes the famous *dhāraṇī* of Śākyamuni expounded in the *Svalpākṣara-prajñāpāramitāsūtra*—"Oṃ mune mune mahāmunaye svāhā"—and this suggests that this maṇḍala evolved from the cult of this *dhāraṇī*. It takes the form of a triple eight-petalled lotus, and Śākyamuni is depicted on the pericarp of the first lotus. On the eight petals of the first lotus are the eight great bodhisattvas Vajrapāṇi, Avalokiteśvara, Mañjuśrī, Ākāśagarbha, Kṣitigarbha, Sarvanīvaraṇaviṣkambhin, Maitreya and Samantabhadra; on the eight petals of the second lotus are eight great *śrāvaka*s; and on the eight petals of the third lotus are the protecters of the ten directions (with two of them outside the lotus). In addition, in the four corners are the four outer offering goddesses, and in the four gates are the four celestial kings. Thus, the total number of deities is thirty-five. Among Mitrayogin's one hundred maṇḍalas, this is the only one taking the form of a triple eight-petalled lotus. It is interesting to note that in Japan the maṇḍala of Buddhalocanā has the same triple eight-petalled lotus. As in the nine-deity Jambhala-maṇḍala (M-5), the colour scheme of the courtyard is that of the Highest Yoga tantras centred on Ratnasambhava (Type G), even though Śākyamuni has no direct connection with Ratnasambhava. This colour scheme may have applied the colours of the four continents in the world system centred on Sumeru to the four quarters of the maṇḍala.

7. Five-deity maṇḍala of White Mañjughoṣa

Pattern: 41b. Four-petalled lotus;
Colour scheme:
Yoga tantras centred
on Vairocana

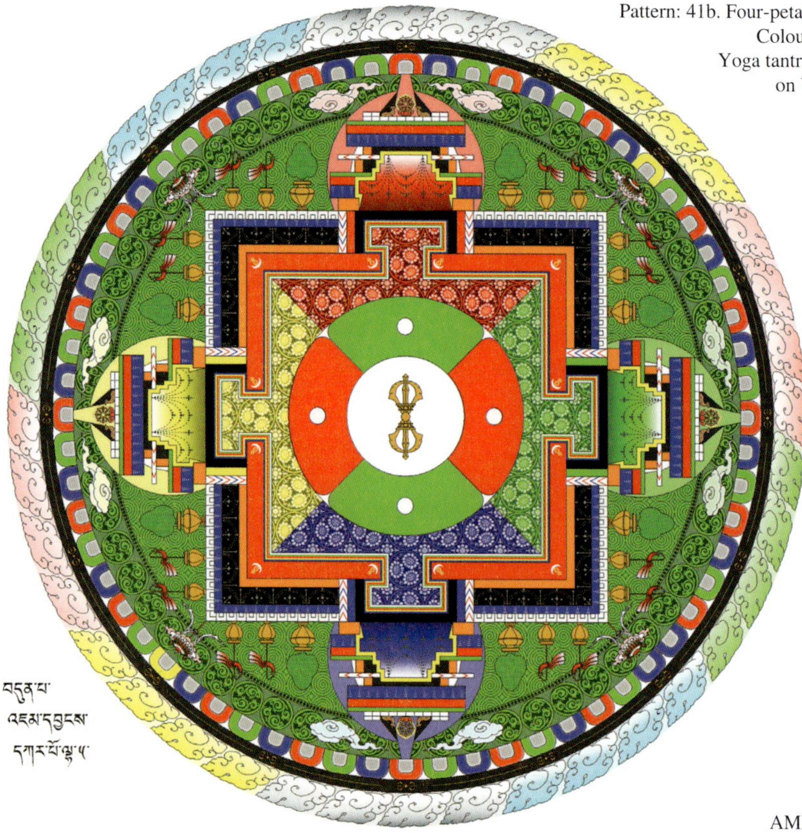

བདུན་པ་
འཇམ་དབྱངས་
དཀར་པོ་ལྷ་ལྔ་

AMM: No. 79

This maṇḍala is centred on Mañjughoṣa/Mañjuśrī, who has the five-syllable mantra "Arapacana." The *Abhisamayamuktāmālā* calls this maṇḍala "Prajñācakra-Arapacana," but the "Prajñācakra-Mañjuśrī-sādhana" in the *Sādhanamālā* (No. 80), which belongs to the Yoga tantras, does not coincide with this maṇḍala. The centre of the maṇḍala takes the form of a four-petalled lotus, on the pericarp of which one-headed and two-armed Mañjuśrī (here represented by a vajra) is depicted, and on the four lotus petals in the cardinal directions are the four attendants Jālinīprabha (east), Candraprabha (south), Keśinī (west) and Upakeśinī (north). The five-syllable mantra corresponds to the five deities of this maṇḍala. These four attendants also appear in the retinue of Mañjuśrī in the Garbhadhātu-maṇḍala of Japanese Esoteric Buddhism. The Ṅor maṇḍalas include the Arapacana-maṇḍala (No. 21), which has the same deities, but it has an eight-petalled lotus rather than a four-petalled lotus, and vases containing nectar (*amṛta*) are arranged in the four intermediate directions. Furthermore, in the Ṅor maṇḍalas the Arapacana-maṇḍala is classified not among the Kriyā tantras but among the Caryā tantras.

8. Thirteen-deity Mahākāruṇika-maṇḍala

Pattern: 36a. Four-petalled lotus;
Colour scheme:
Yoga tantras centred
on Amitābha

བརྒྱད་པ་ཐུགས་རྗེ་ཆེན་
པོ་ལྷ་༡༣་

AMM: No. 7

In Tibet, Mahākāruṇika (Thugs rje chen po) often signifies the eleven-headed and eight-armed form of Avalokiteśvara revealed by the nun Lakṣmī. However, this Mahākāruṇika-maṇḍala is centred on four-armed Avalokiteśvara described in the *Kāraṇḍavyūha-sūtra*. The *Kāraṇḍavyūha-sūtra* explains the renowned six-syllable mantra of Avalokiteśvara ("Oṃ maṇi padme hūṃ") and is considered to be the basic scripture of the Avalokiteśvara cult in Tibet and Nepal. The centre of the maṇḍala takes the form of a four-petalled lotus, with Maṇidhara and Muktādhara on the petals flanking the main deity and dBaṅ gi rgyal po (Sanskrit name unknown) and Āryāvalokiteśvara on the petals in front and behind. In the four corners are the four outer offering goddesses, and in the four gates are the four female gatekeepers Aṅkuśī, Pāśī, Sphoṭā and Ghaṇṭā. Thus, this maṇḍala consists of thirteen deities. The colour scheme of the courtyard is that of the Yoga tantras centred on Amitābha (Type B) since Avalokiteśvara, the main deity, belongs to the Lotus family presided over by Amitābha. This maṇḍala can be interpreted as a development of the triad consisting of Amitāyus (four-armed Avalokiteśvara in this case), Maṇidhara and Ṣaḍakṣarī expounded in the *Kāraṇḍavyūha-sūtra*. The Ṅor maṇḍalas, on the other hand, include a Cintāmaṇi-Jagaḍḍāmara-maṇḍala attributed to Sroṅ btsan sgam po (No. 130), which is centred on the same four-armed Avalokiteśvara. However, there are very few examples of either of these maṇḍalas in Tibet.

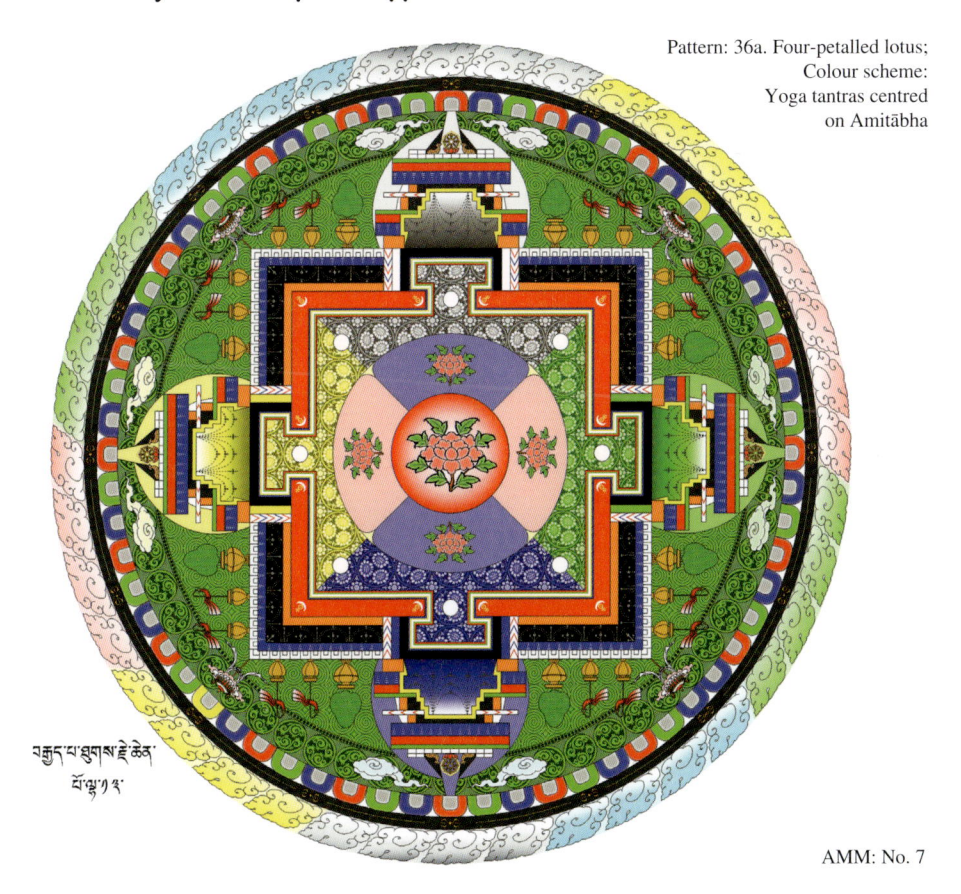

9. Five-deity Amoghapāśa-maṇḍala

Pattern: 48. Four-spoked wheel;
Colour scheme:
Yoga tantras centred
on Vairocana

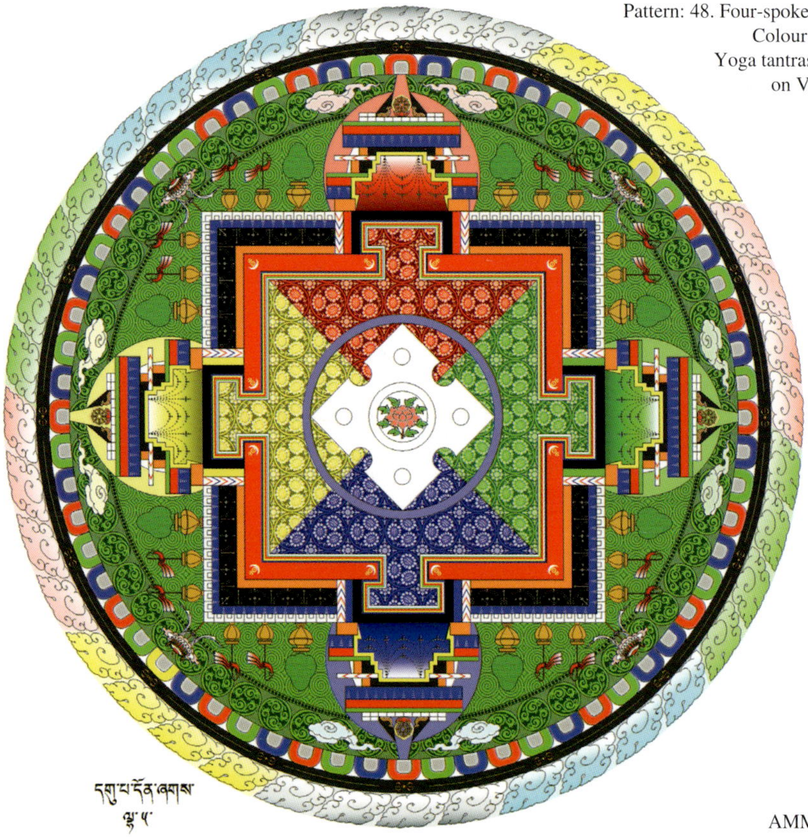

དགུ་པ་དོན་ཞགས་
ལྔ་པ་

AMM: No. 90

The Amoghapāśa pentad (*Don źags lha lṅa*) is a selection of the principal deities described in the *Amoghapāśa-kalparāja*, and in Tibet several combinations are known. Among these, the most popular is that centred on one-headed and two-armed Avalokiteśvara accompanied by the four attendants Amoghapāśa (east), Hayagrīva (south), Ekajaṭā (west) and Bhṛkuṭī (north). The *Abhisamayamuktāmālā* explains a maṇḍala of the same pentad, although the main deity is called Khasarpaṇi. The Ṅor maṇḍalas, on the other hand, include a sixteen-deity Amoghapāśa-maṇḍala (No. 12) which adds a further eleven attendants. In addition, several examples of five-deity Amoghapāśa maṇḍalas have been discovered in the Mogao Caves near Dunhuang. This fact suggests that the Amoghapāśa pentad was revered from the eighth to tenth centuries in India and along the Silk Road. All of these examples add attendant deities. The present maṇḍala, on the other hand, has a simple structure with Avalokiteśvara (here represented by a lotus) and four attendants on a four-spoked wheel. In Tibet, the Amoghapāśa pentad also takes the form of a group of statues, a representative example of which is found in the Amoghapāśa Chapel (Don źags lha khang) on the west side of the second floor of the Great Stūpa of dPal 'khor chos sde in rGyal rtse.

10. Five-deity Siṃhanāda-maṇḍala

Pattern: 47. Four-petalled lotus;
Colour scheme:
Yoga tantras centred
on Vairocana

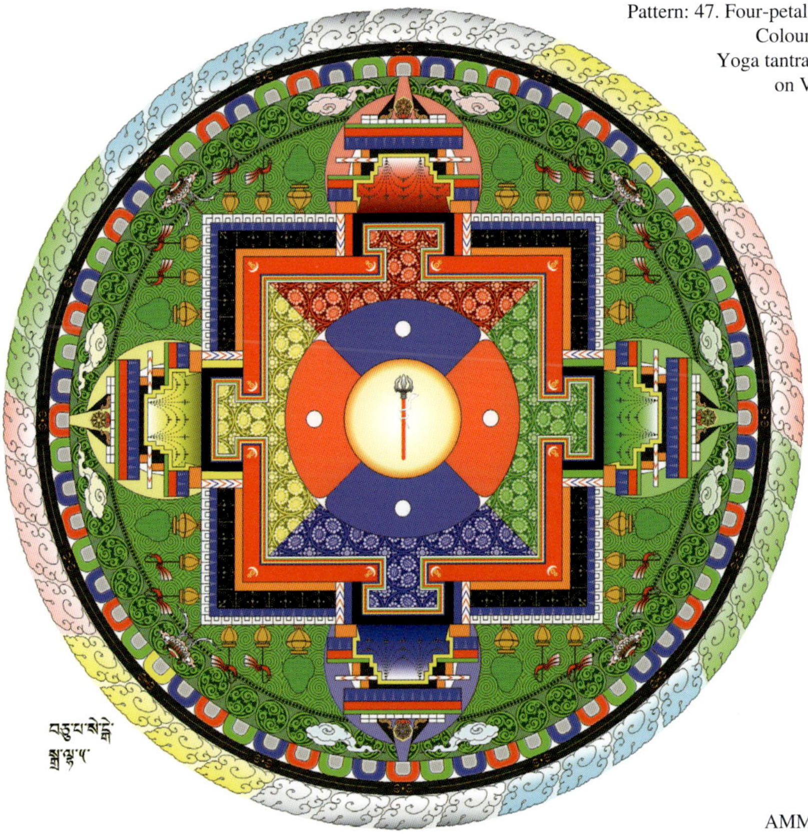

AMM: No. 89

Siṃhanāda is a transformation of Avalokiteśvara, one-headed and two-armed and riding on a lion in a posture of royal ease. Several fine images of Siṃhanāda have been unearthed in India. However, he was not transmitted to the Sino-Japanese tradition of Buddhism because his cult came into existence only in the ninth century. In Tibet, he was regarded as a deity who subjugates *nāga*s, and his *dhāraṇī* was believed to be effective against serious diseases. It is interesting that the symbol of this deity, a trident around which a white snake is entwined, is somewhat similar to the rod of Asclepius, the symbol of medicine in the West. In particular, leprosy, which was feared by Tibetans, was believed to be due to the curse of some evil *nāga*, and consequently Siṃhanāda was the object of special devotion to prevent leprosy. In this maṇḍala, a snake-entwined trident, the symbol of this deity, is depicted on the pericarp of the four-petalled lotus, and four Buddhas are arranged on the lotus petals in the cardinal directions. The colour scheme of the courtyard ought to be that of the Yoga tantras centred on Amitābha since the *Abhisamayamuktāmālā* explains that Vairocana should be depicted in the west where Amitābha is usually located. However, the Hahn Foundation handscroll adopts that of the Yoga tantras centred on Vairocana.

11. Seventeen-deity Hayagrīva-maṇḍala

Pattern: 49a. Eight-spoked wheel;
Colour scheme:
Highest Yoga tantras
centred on Akṣobhya

AMM: No. 6

This maṇḍala is centred on two-armed Hayagrīva, who holds a club made of acacia in his right hand and forms the *tarjanī-mudrā* with his left hand. The Sino-Japanese tradition of Mahāyāna Buddhism classifies Hayagrīva as one of the transformations of Avalokiteśvara, but in Tibet he is classified as a wrathful deity even though he is thought to be an emanation of Avalokiteśvara. According to the *Abhisamayamuktāmālā*, this maṇḍala takes the form of an eight-spoked wheel, in the centre of which Hayagrīva (here represented by a club) is depicted. On the spokes of the wheel are the eight wrathful deities Vijaya (east), Nīladaṇḍa (southeast), Yamāntaka (south), Acala (southwest), Mahāhūṃ (west), Ṭakkirāja (northwest), Amṛtakuṇḍalin (north) and Trailokyavijaya (northeast). In the four corners of the courtyard are the four outer offering goddesses Dhūpā, Puṣpā, Dīpā and Gandhā, and in the four gates are the four gatekeepers Vajrāṅkuśa, Vajrapāśa, Vajrasphoṭa and Vajrāveśa. Thus, the total number of deities is seventeen. The colour scheme of the courtyard ought to be centred on Amitābha since Hayagrīva belongs to the Lotus family presided over by Amitābha. However, the Hahn Foundation handscroll adopts that of the Highest Yoga tantras centred on Akṣobhya. The Ṅor maṇḍalas include several maṇḍalas of Hayagrīva, but none of them is identical with this maṇḍala. No coloured thangka depicting this maṇḍala has been identified to date.

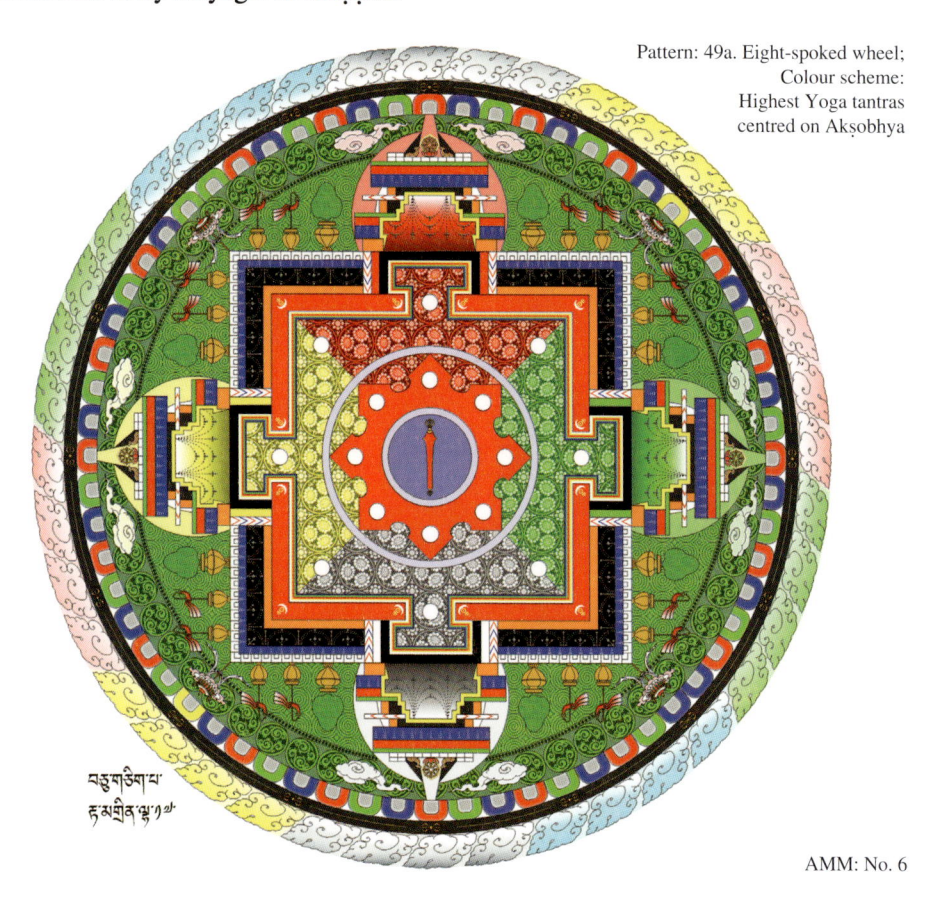

12. Eleven-deity Acala-maṇḍala

Pattern: 36b. Four-petalled lotus;
Colour scheme:
Highest Yoga tantras
centred on Akṣobhya

བཅུ་གཉིས་པ་
མི་གཡོ་བ་ལྷ་༡༡་

AMM: No. 81

This maṇḍala is centred on Acala, blue-black in colour, who holds a sword made of crystal in his right hand and forms the *tarjanī-mudrā* with his left hand while holding a noose. *Roṅ tha's Iconometry* explains the form of this maṇḍala as a four-petalled lotus, while the *Abhisamayamuktāmālā* describes a ten-spoked wheel, and the Hahn Foundation handscroll coincides with the latter. Acala (here represented by a sword) is depicted on the hub of the wheel, and on the ten spokes are ten wrathful deities. The *Abhisamayamuktāmālā* does not give the names of these ten wrathful deities, but in many cases they are the ten wrathful deities mentioned in the *Guhyasamāja-tantra*. However, the ten wrathful deities of the *Guhyasamāja-tantra* include Acala, and consequently Acala is duplicated. In the seventeen-deity Hayagrīva-maṇḍala (M-11), the name of the wrathful deity in west, who is the same as the main deity, has been changed to Mahāhūṃ. In this maṇḍala too the name of the wrathful deity in the southwest may also have been changed. There are several opinions regarding the affiliation of Acala. As for the colour scheme of the courtyard, the Hahn Foundation handscroll adopts that of the Highest Yoga tantras centred on Akṣobhya on the assumption that Acala belongs to the Vajra family presided over by Akṣobhya. The Ṅor maṇḍalas include a nine-deity Acala maṇḍala (No. 48), but it belongs to the Highest Yoga tantras and differs from this maṇḍala.

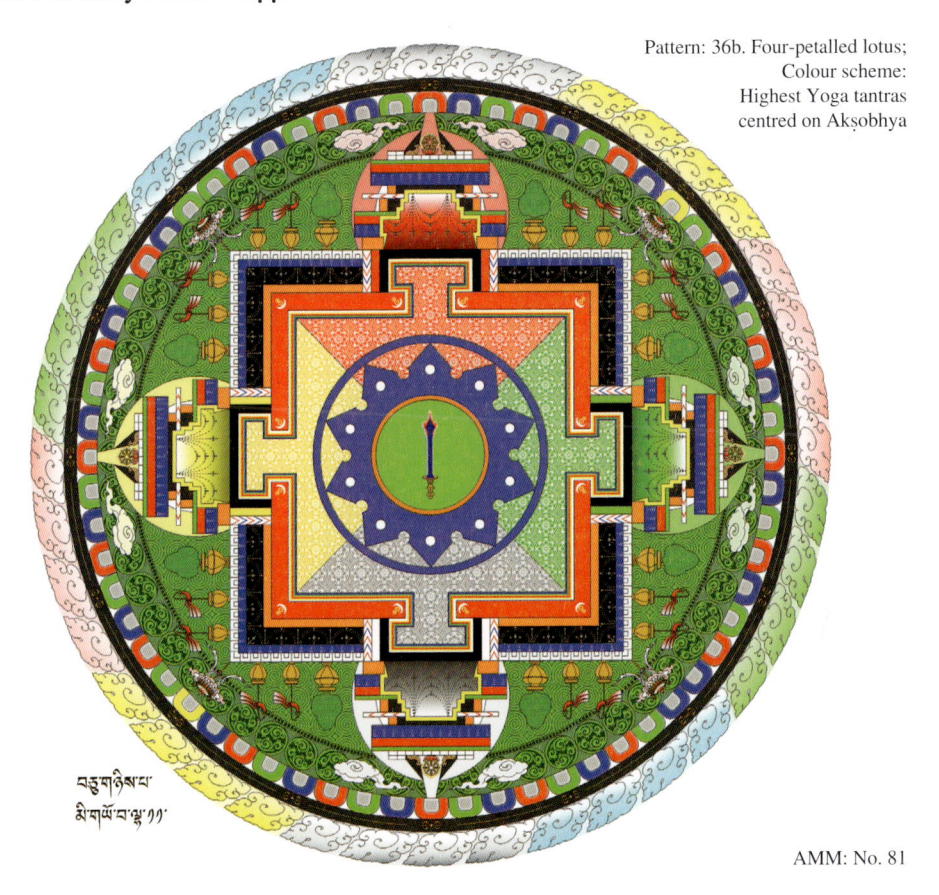

13. Twenty-three-deity Vajravidāraṇa-maṇḍala

Pattern: 39. Four-spoked wheel;
Colour scheme:
Highest Yoga tantras
centred on Akṣobhya

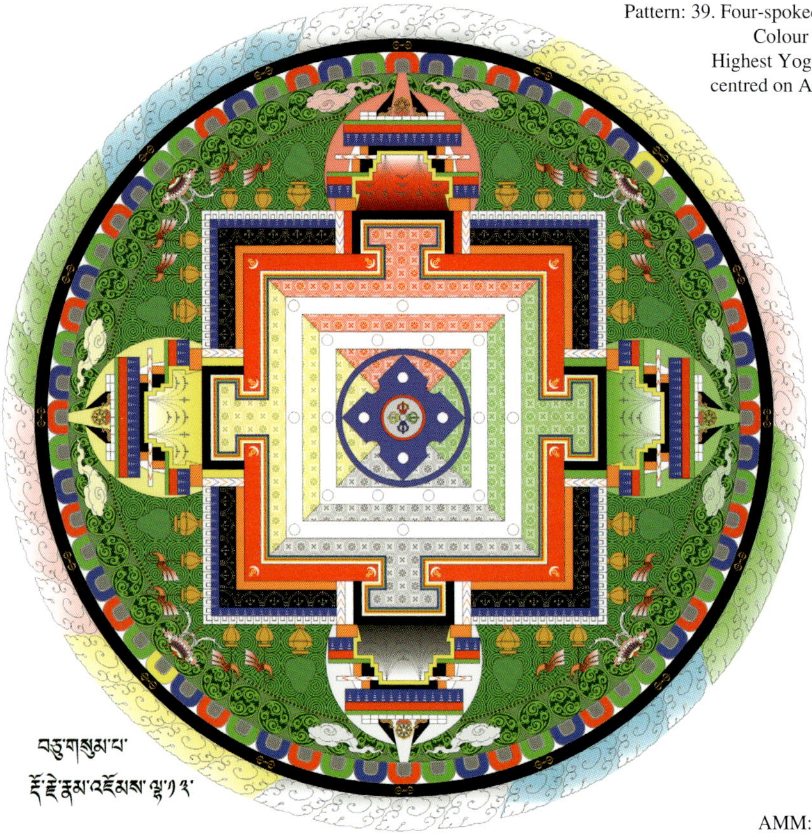

བཅུ་གསུམ་པ་
རྡོ་རྗེ་རྣམ་འཇོམས་ལྷ་༡༣་

AMM: No. 103

Vajravidāraṇa is a deification of the *Vajravidāraṇī-dhāraṇī,* a *dhāraṇī* centred on Vajrapāṇi. Although this *dhāraṇī* is not popular in Sino-Japanese Esoteric Buddhism, it was widely recited in Tibet from the time of the Tufan kingdom. Various forms of this deity are known in Tibet, and this maṇḍala is centred on a wrathful form that is green in colour and holds a crossed vajra in his right hand and draws a vajra-bell towards his body with his left hand, which forms the *tarjanī-mudrā*. This maṇḍala takes the form of a four-spoked wheel, and on the spokes in the four cardinal directions are Vajracaṇḍa (east; reading *gtum po* for *rtum po* in the *Abhisamayamuktā-mālā*), Vajrakīla (south), Vajradaṇḍa (west) and Vajramudgara (north). This four-spoked wheel is surrounded by a double square: in the first square are the protectors of the ten directions and in the second square the goddesses of the eight auspicious signs (*bkra śis rtags brgyad*). The goddesses of the eight auspicious signs seem to be the same as the eight attendants in the thirteen-deity Akṣobhya-maṇḍala (M-21). Thus, the total number of deities is twenty-three, but the inscription on the Hahn Foundation handscroll makes it thirteen. However, this would seem to be an error since the number of seats for the deities in the handscroll is twenty-three. The colour scheme of the courtyard is that of the Highest Yoga tantras centred on Akṣobhya (Type E) since Vajravidāraṇa is an emanation of Vajrapāṇi.

14. Nine-deity Vajrapāṇi-maṇḍala

Pattern: 48. Four-spoked wheel;
Colour scheme:
Highest Yoga tantras
centred on Akṣobhya

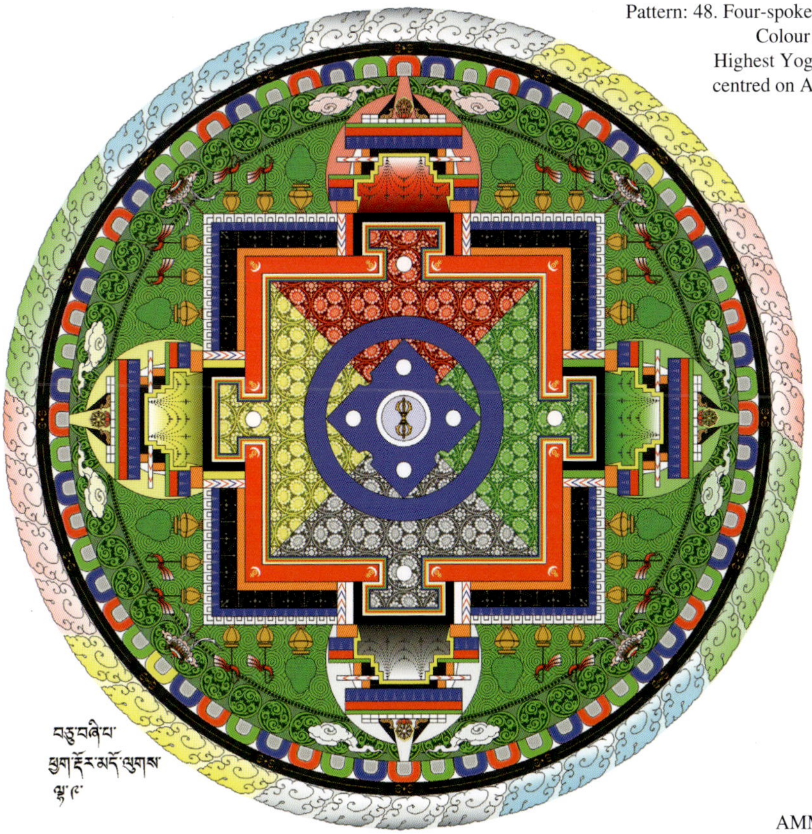

བཅུ་བཞི་པ་
ཕྱག་རྡོར་མདོ་ལུགས
ལྷ་༩

AMM: No. 2

According to the *Abhisamayamuktāmālā*, this maṇḍala was devised by Ācārya Nāgārjuna in accordance with a sūtra and a *dhāraṇī*. The Tibetan Tripiṭaka includes a ritual manual entitled *Vajrapāṇi-maṇḍala-vidhi* (Peking No. 3712) attributed to Nāgārjuna, and this is thought to be the textual source of this maṇḍala. It takes the form of a four-spoked wheel, on the hub of which one-headed and two armed Vajrapāṇi-Guhyakādhipati, holding a vajra in his right hand and forming the *tarjanī-mudrā* with his left hand, is depicted as the main deity. On the spokes in the four cardinal directions are Vajrayakṣa (east), Vajrarākṣasa (south), Vajramahāgraha (west) and Vajravetāla (north), and in the four gates are the four female gatekeepers Aṅkuśī, Pāśī, Sphoṭā and Ghaṇṭā. As in other maṇḍalas centred on Vajrapāṇi, the colour scheme of the courtyard is that of the Highest Yoga tantras centred on Akṣobhya (Type E). This maṇḍala is not included in any other maṇḍala sets, nor has any coloured thangka depicting this maṇḍala been identified. However, Sūtrakrama-Vajrapāṇi (Phyag rdor rdo lugs), corresponding to the main deity of this maṇḍala, is included in the *Five Hundred Gods of Narthang*.

15. Single-deity Vajrapāṇi-maṇḍala

Pattern: 47. Four-petalled lotus;
Colour scheme:
Highest Yoga tantras
centred on Akṣobhya

བཅོ་ལྔ་པ་
ཕྱག་རྡོར་བདུད་ཐིག་
ལྔ་ཀ་

AMM: No. 83

According to the *Abhisamayamuktāmālā*, the maṇḍala of Vajrapāṇi "Drop of Amṛta" takes the form of a four-petalled lotus. It is a single-deity maṇḍala centred on three-headed and six-armed Vajrapāṇi (here represented by a vajra). The main deity Vajrapāṇi holds snakes with two of his six hands and is devouring them. This means that this special style of Vajrapāṇi was thought to be a subjugator of evil *nāga*s. It is not explained in the text why this maṇḍala is called "Drop of Amṛta" (bDud rtsi thig pa). However, the *Abhisamayamuktāmālā* explains that one should meditate on four vajras symbolizing the five wisdoms in the four cardinal directions around the main deity. The four white circles inside yellow ovals depicted in the Hahn Foundation handscroll seem to be four minute vajras inside drops of *amṛta*. As in other maṇḍalas centred on Vajrapāṇi, the colour scheme of the courtyard is that of the Highest Yoga tantras centred on Akṣobhya (Type E). This maṇḍala is not included in any other maṇḍala sets, nor has any coloured thangka depicting this maṇḍala been identified. The main deity Vajrapāṇi "Drop of Amṛta" is also not found in any other compendia of iconography apart from those which bring together all the main deities of Mitrayogin's 108 maṇḍalas. Thus, the cult of this deity would seem to have been rather limited in Tibet.

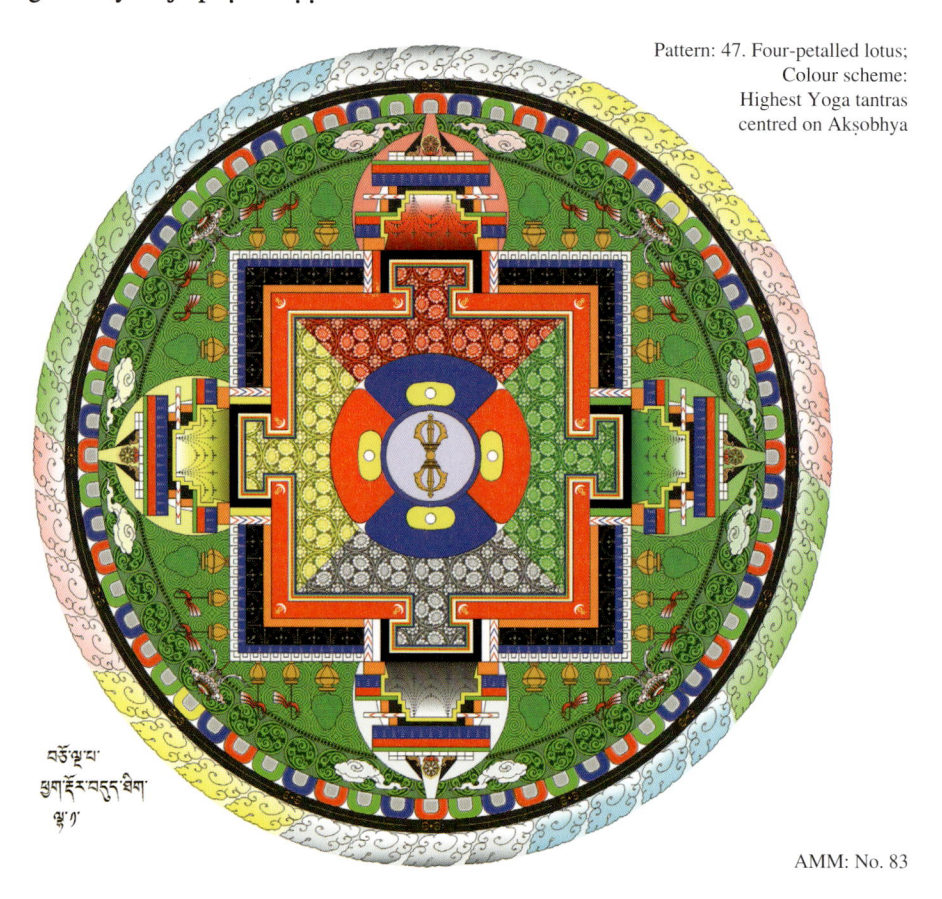

16. Single-deity Nīlāmbaradharavajrapāṇi-maṇḍala

Pattern: 49b. Eight-petalled lotus;
Colour scheme:
Highest Yoga tantras
centred on Akṣobhya

བཅུ་དྲུག་པ་
ཕྱག་རྡོར་གོས་
སྔོན་ཅན་ལྷ་ ༡

AMM: No. 84

Nīlāmbaradharavajrapāṇi, or "Vajrapāṇi Clad in a Blue Garment," is one of the transformations of Vajrapāṇi found mainly in the Kriyā tantras. As is indicated by the fact that the *Abhisamayamuktāmālā* characterizes this maṇḍala as *mdor bsdus pa* (condensed), it is one of the simpler maṇḍalas among the maṇḍalas centred on Nīlāmbaradharavajrapāṇi. It depicts one-headed and two armed Nīlāmbaradharavajrapāṇi (here represented by a vajra) holding a vajra in his right hand and forming the *tarjanī-mudrā* with his left hand on the pericarp of an eight-petalled lotus. On the surrounding eight petals is inscribed in Tibetan script the character "Hūṃ," which is frequently used as the seed-syllable of wrathful deities. According to the *Abhisamayamuktāmālā,* this maṇḍala takes the form of a four-petalled lotus, while *Roṅ tha's Iconometry* makes it an eight-petalled lotus, as does the Hahn Foundation handscroll. While stating that this maṇḍala takes the form of a four-petalled lotus, the *Abhisamayamuktāmālā* also explains that one should visualize the letter "Hūṃ" on eight petals, and so there appears to be some inconsistency in its explanation. Mitrayogin's intention may have been to visualize nine four-petalled lotuses and arrange the main deity and eight "Hūṃ" letters on the pericarps of the lotuses. As in other maṇḍalas centred on Vajrapāṇi, the colour scheme of the courtyard is that of the Highest Yoga tantras centred on Akṣobhya (Type E).

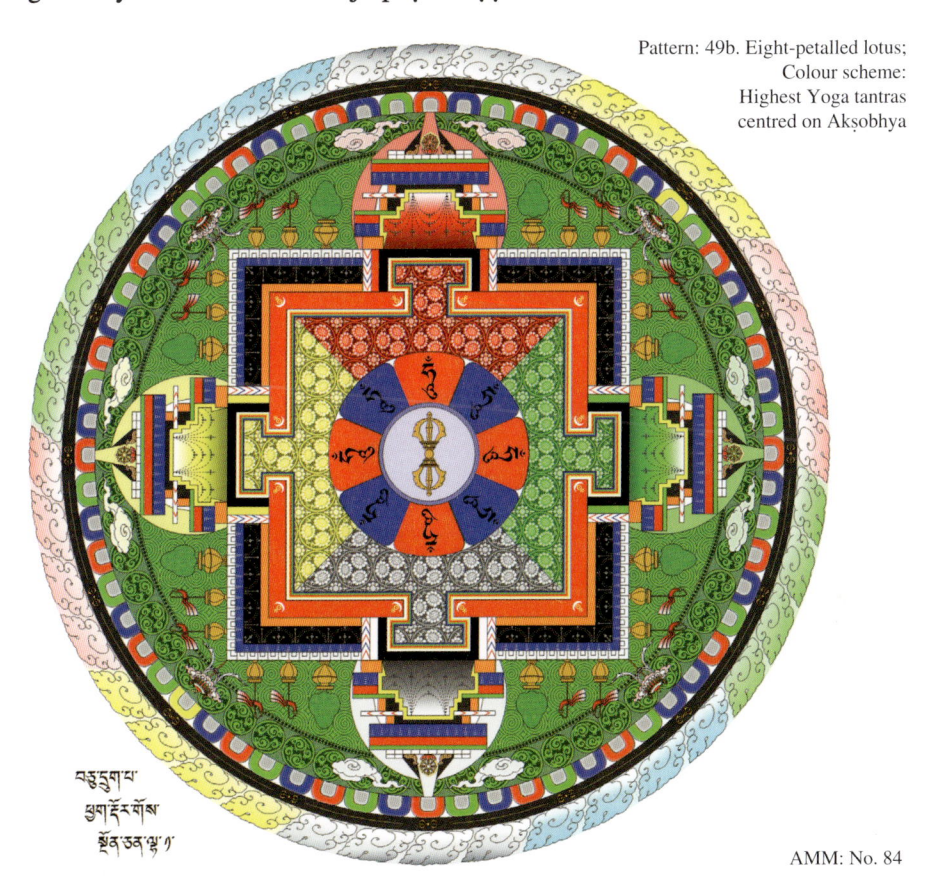

17. Five-stūpa Vajrapāṇi-maṇḍala

Pattern: 47. Four-petalled lotus;
Colour scheme:
Highest Yoga tantras
centred on Akṣobhya

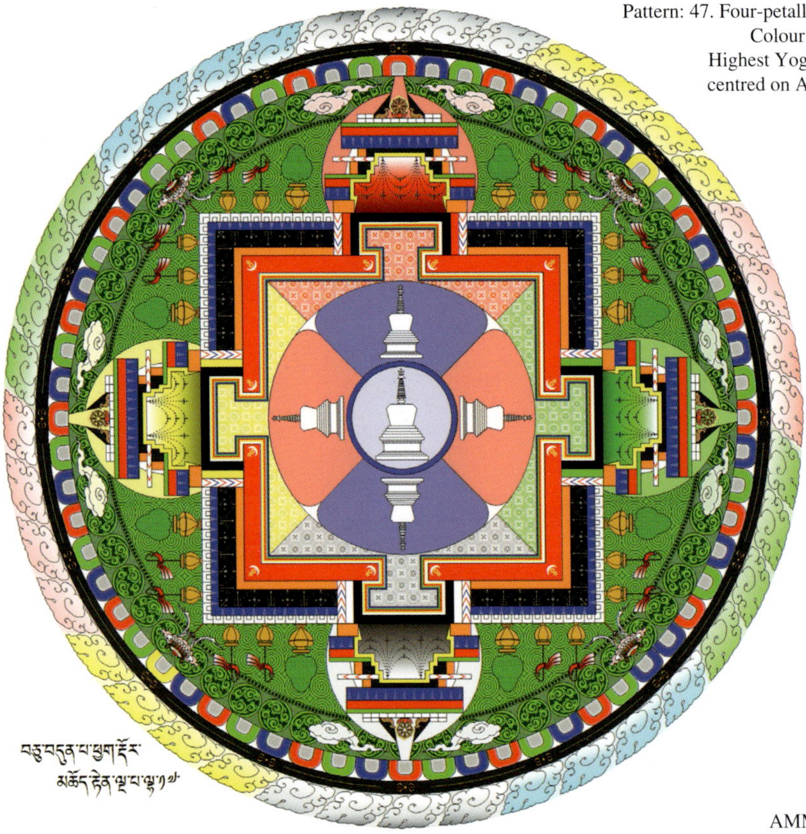

AMM: No. 85

According to the *Abhisamayamuktāmālā,* this maṇḍala takes the form of a four-petalled lotus. On the pericarp and four petals of the lotus one should visualize five stūpas, and in the centre stands Vajrapāṇi, blue in colour and in the *ālīḍha* posture (with the right leg stretched out and the left leg bent), holding a vajra in his right hand and a bell in his left hand. Moreover, Indra is emerging from his right armpit and Sūrya from his left armpit, both holding a vajra and a bell, the attributes of Vajrapāṇi (reading *bteg pa* for *rteg pa* in the *Abhisamayamuktāmālā*). Inside the stūpas in the four cardinal directions are Vairocana (east), Ratnasambhava (south), Amitābha (west) and Amoghasiddhi (north). The *Abhisamayamuktāmālā* and *Roṅ tha's Iconometry* call this maṇḍala "Blue Stūpa"(*mchod rten sṅon po*). However, the inscription on the Hahn Foundation handscroll reads "having five stūpas" (*mchod rten lṅa pa*), and judging from the pictorial representation of this maṇḍala this would seem to be more appropriate. In Nepal there still exist such sets of five stūpas, collectively symbolizing the five Buddhas. The colour scheme of the courtyard is that of the Highest Yoga tantras centred on Akṣobhya (Type E), which coincides with the arrangement of the five Buddhas in this maṇḍala. This maṇḍala is not included in any other maṇḍala sets, nor has any coloured thangka depicting this maṇḍala been identified.

18. Thirteen-deity Vajrapāṇi-maṇḍala

Pattern: 48. Four-spoked wheel;
Colour scheme:
Highest Yoga tantras
centred on Akṣobhya

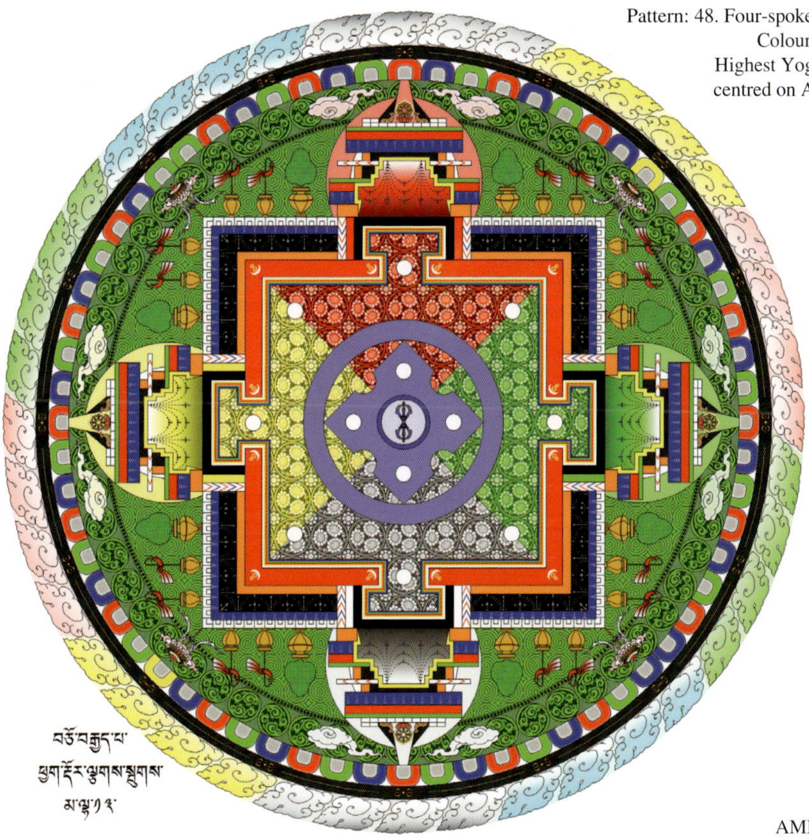

བཅོ་བརྒྱད་པ་
ཕྱག་རྡོར་ལྕགས་སྦུགས་
མ་ལྷ་༡༣་

AMM: No. 3

According to the *Abhisamayamuktāmālā*, this maṇḍala is centred on one-headed and four-armed Vajrapāṇi, who brandishes a sword with his principal right hand, holds a bell in his principal left hand, and devours a snake with his remaining two hands. Vajrapāṇi's head reaches the paradise of Paranirmitavaśavartin while his legs touch the bottom of the ocean, and he makes Mount Meru his seat. Thus, this Vajrapāṇi is visualized as a being of tremendous size. This maṇḍala takes the form of a four-spoked wheel, in the centre of which the main deity (here represented by a vajra) is depicted, and Vajrapāṇis of the four families—Tathāgata family (east), Jewel family (south), Lotus family (west) and Action family (north)—are arranged on the spokes in the four cardinal directions. Four *garuḍa*s of the four families, who devour snakes, are in the four corners, and in the four gates are the four gatekeepers Vajrāṅkuśa, Vajrapāśa, Vajrasphoṭa and Vajrāveśa. As in other maṇḍalas centred on Vajrapāṇi, the colour scheme of the courtyard is that of the Highest Yoga tantras centred on Akṣobhya (Type E). This maṇḍala is rarely included in other maṇḍala sets, nor has any coloured thangka depicting this maṇḍala been identified. In addition, the reason for the strange designation "Iron Pipe/Key" (lCags sbugs ma) for the main deity is not clear.

19. Five-deity Garuḍa-Vajrapāṇi-maṇḍala

Pattern: 48. Four-spoked wheel;
Colour scheme:
Highest Yoga tantras
centred on Akṣobhya

བཅུ་དགུ་པ་
ཕྱག་རྡོར་གཏུམ་པོ་
ཁྱུང་ཤོ་ཅན་ལྷ་༥་

AMM: No. 86

According to the *Abhisamayamuktāmālā* and *Roṅ tha's Iconometry,* the main deity of this maṇḍala is "rDo rje gtum po khyuṅ gśam can" (wrathful vajra with the lower half of the body of a *garuḍa*). The inscription of the Hahn Foundation handscroll, on the other hand, reads "Phyag rdor gtum po khyuṅ śo can" (Vajrapāṇi with a row of *garuḍa*s), which should probably read "Phyag rdor gtum po khyuṅ gśog can" (Vajrapāṇi with the wing of a *garuḍa*). This maṇḍala takes the form of a four-spoked wheel, on the hub of which is the main deity, one-headed and two-armed Garuḍa-Vajrapāṇi (here represented by a vajra), who brandishes a vajra with his right hand and forms the *tarjanī-mudrā* with his left hand. A *garuḍa* emerges from his left hand forming the *tarjanī-mudrā*, and this is a distinctive characteristic of the main deity. The four wrathful deities Vijaya (east), Yamāntaka (south), Hayagrīva (west) and Amṛtakuṇḍalin (north) are arranged on the spokes in the four cardinal directions. As in other maṇḍalas centred on Vajrapāṇi, the colour scheme of the courtyard is that of the Highest Yoga tantras centred on Akṣobhya (Type E). This maṇḍala is not included in any other maṇḍala sets, nor has any coloured thangka depicting this maṇḍala been identified.

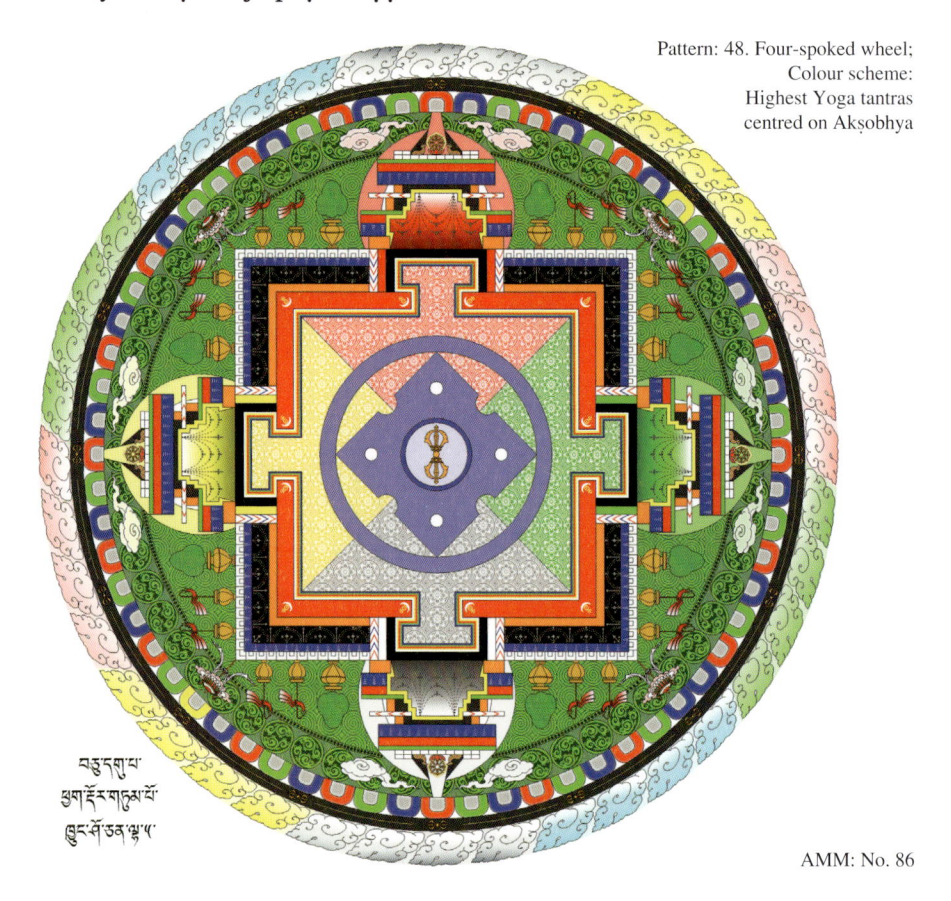

20. Nine-deity Vajragaruḍa-maṇḍala

Pattern: 49a. Eight-spoked wheel;
Colour scheme:
Highest Yoga tantras
centred on Akṣobhya

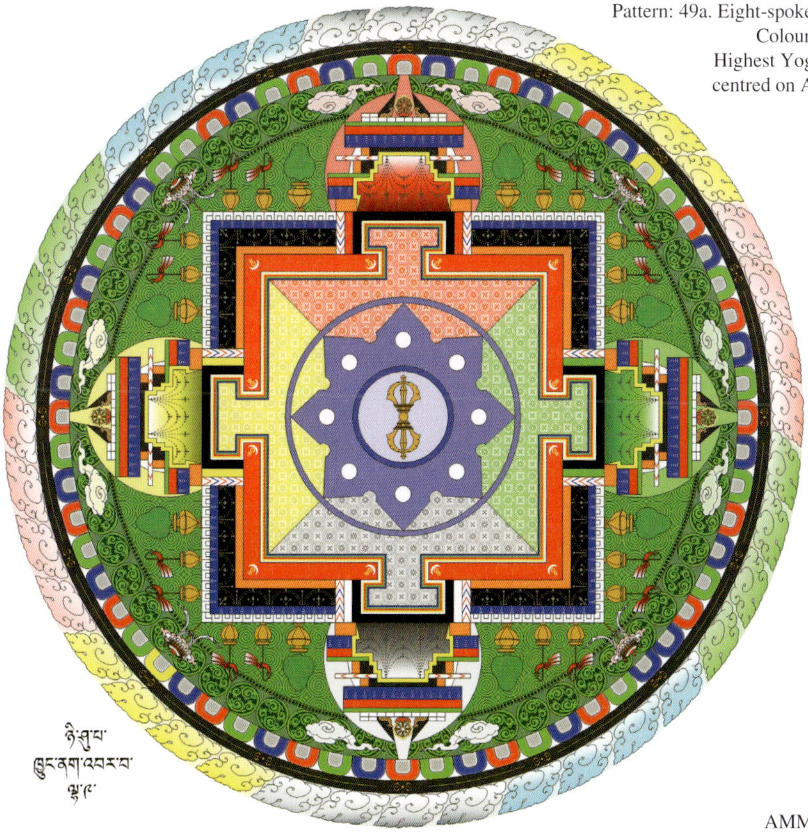

ཉི་ཤུ་པ་
ཁྱུང་ནག་འབར་བ་
ལྷ་༩་

AMM: No. 87

Vajragaruḍa is a deification of the *garuḍa*, an imaginary bird that eats *nāga*s, or serpents, and he is mainly worshipped as a deity who subjugates *nāga*s. According to the *Abhisamayamuktāmālā*, his body combines parts of six kinds of animals, namely, the horns of female yaks, the eyes of frogs, the lips of sheep (reading *mtshul pa* for *'tshul pa*), the hands of human beings, the wings of birds, and the nails of fierce animals. This maṇḍala takes the form of an eight-spoked wheel, on the hub of which Vajragaruḍa devouring a snake (here represented by a vajra) is depicted as the main deity. On the eight spokes in the four cardinal and four intermediate directions are Vajragaruḍa (east), a club (southeast), a jewel (south), a hammer (southwest), a lotus (west), a sword (northwest), a crossed vajra (north) and a chopper with a fearsome *garuḍa* (northeast). (The directions are not mentioned in the text and are conjectural.) As in other maṇḍalas centred on a wrathful deity belonging to the Vajra family, the colour scheme of the courtyard is that of the Highest Yoga tantras centred on Akṣobhya (Type E). This maṇḍala is not included in any other maṇḍala sets. However, an image of Vajragaruḍa, the main deity, is included in the *Three Hundred Icons* and *Three Hundred and Sixty Icons* (*Eulogies to Sacred Images of Buddhas and Bodhisattvas*), and he seems to have been worshipped as an independent deity.

21. Thirteen-deity Akṣobhya-maṇḍala

Pattern: 36b. Four-petalled lotus;
Colour scheme:
Highest Yoga tantras
centred on Akṣobhya

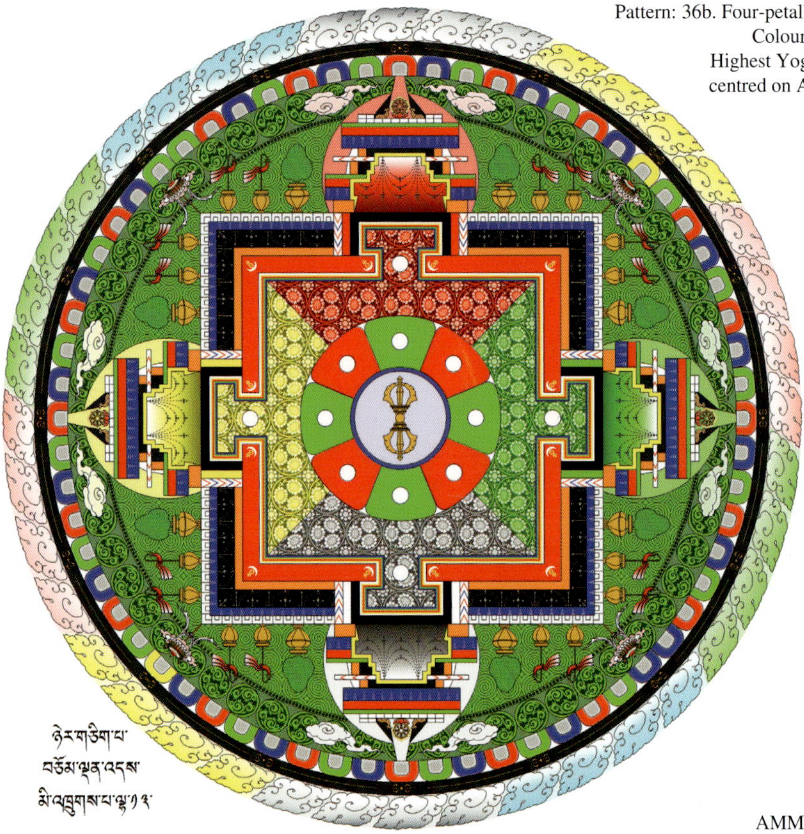

ཉེར་གཅིག་པ་
བཅོམ་ལྡན་འདས་
མི་འཁྲུགས་པ་ལྷ་༡༣་

AMM: No. 101

Akṣobhya is the Buddha of the realm of Abhirati (Delight) in the east and is worshipped as a typical Buddha of another world-realm along with Amitābha of the realm of Sukhāvatī in the west. This maṇḍala is centred on Akṣobhya (here represented by a vajra), and surrounding him are eight goddesses who symbolize the eight auspicious signs (*bkra śis rtags brgyad*): the unending string (*śrī-vatsa*), the wheel of the Law (*dharma-cakra*), the lotus, the victorious banner, the parasol, the flask, the white conch-shell and the goldfish. There are two types of Akṣobhya-maṇḍala: in one the eight auspicious signs are arranged around the main deity, and in the other they are depicted as goddesses holding the corresponding auspicious sign. The Ṅor maṇḍalas contain two types of nine-deity Akṣobhya-maṇḍala, with that transmitted by Atīśa (No. 14) being centred on Akṣobhya as the *sambhogakāya* and that transmitted by Śavarī (No. 15) being centred on Akṣobhya as the *nirmāṇakāya*. The present example adds the four female gatekeepers Aṅkuśī, Pāśī, Sphoṭā and Ghanṭā, making a total of thirteen deities. According to *Roṅ tha's Iconometry*, this maṇḍala takes the form of a four-petalled lotus like the thirteen-deity Mahākāruṇika-maṇḍala (M-8), while the *Abhisamayamuktāmālā* makes it an eight-petalled lotus, and many exemplars, including the Hahn Foundation handscroll, coincide with this latter prescription. Many examples of this maṇḍala were produced and have survived in Tibet and Nepal since it was thought to be effective for washing away the sins of a deceased person.

22. Seventeen-deity Vajrapāṇi-maṇḍala (as transmitted by Sugatigarbha)

Pattern: 38. Eight-spoked wheel;
Colour scheme:
Highest Yoga tantras
centred on Akṣobhya

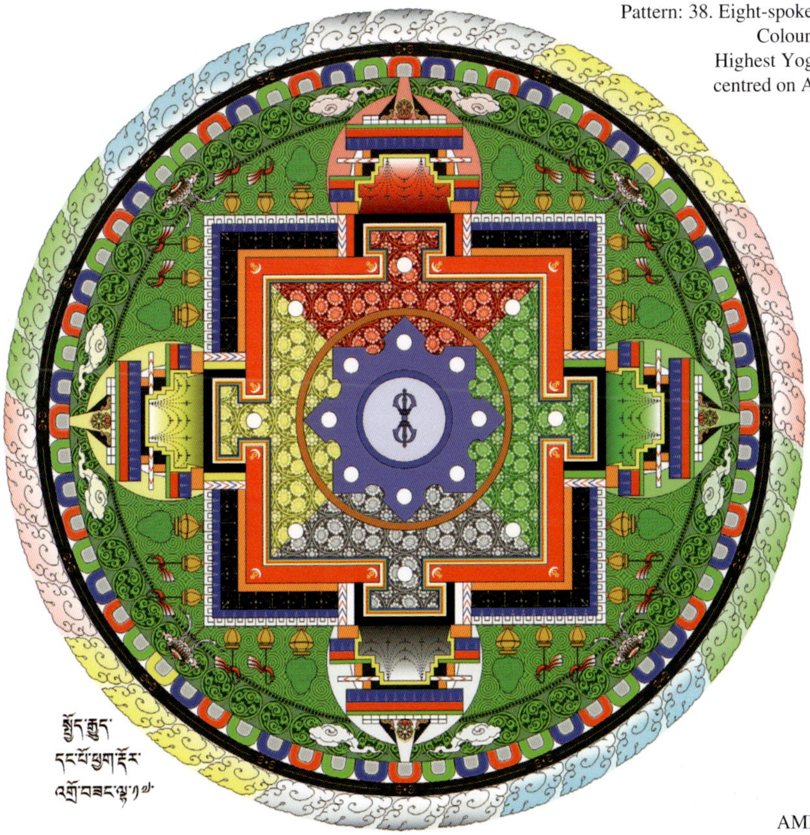

སྤྱོད་རྒྱུད་
དང་པོ་ཕྱག་རྡོར་
འགྲོ་བཟང་ལྷ་༡༧

AMM: No. 1

Sugatigarbha, an Indian practitioner of Esoteric Buddhism, wrote many ritual manuals relating to Nīlāmbaradharavajrapāṇi, or "Vajrapāṇi Clad in Blue Garments," and in Tibet the form of Vajrapāṇi based on his manuals was called the "Sugatigarbha tradition" (*'Gro bzaṅ lugs*). In the *Abhisamayamuktāmālā*, this maṇḍala is placed at the very beginning, and this suggests that Mitrayogin attached some importance to this tradition. It takes the form of an eight-spoked wheel, on the hub of which Vajrapāṇi (here represented by a vajra) is depicted. On the spokes in the four cardinal and four intermediate directions are eight wrathful deities starting with Vajramahābala (east), in the four corners are the four outer offering goddesses Puṣpā, Dhūpā, Dīpā and Gandhā, and in the four gates are the four gatekeepers Vajrāṅkuśa, Vajrapāśa, Vajrasphoṭa and Vajrāveśa. In addition, the *Abhisamayamuktāmālā* mentions twenty great *yakṣa*s and thirty-two wrathful Dharma-protecting deities. However, the Hahn Foundation handscroll neither depicts these nor includes them in the number of deities. The Ṅor maṇḍalas also include a Vajrapāṇi-maṇḍala as transmitted by Sugatigarbha (No. 19), but it is classified among the Kriyā tantras rather than the Caryā tantras. Although this maṇḍala belongs to the Caryā tantras, the colour scheme of the courtyard is that of the Highest Yoga tantras centred on Akṣobhya (Type E) since it is centred on Vajrapāṇi, who belongs to the Vajra family presided over by Akṣobhya.

23. One-hundred-and-five-deity Sarvavid-Vairocana-maṇḍala

Pattern: Nine-panel grid + sixteen-spoked wheel;
Colour scheme: Yoga tantras centred on Vairocana

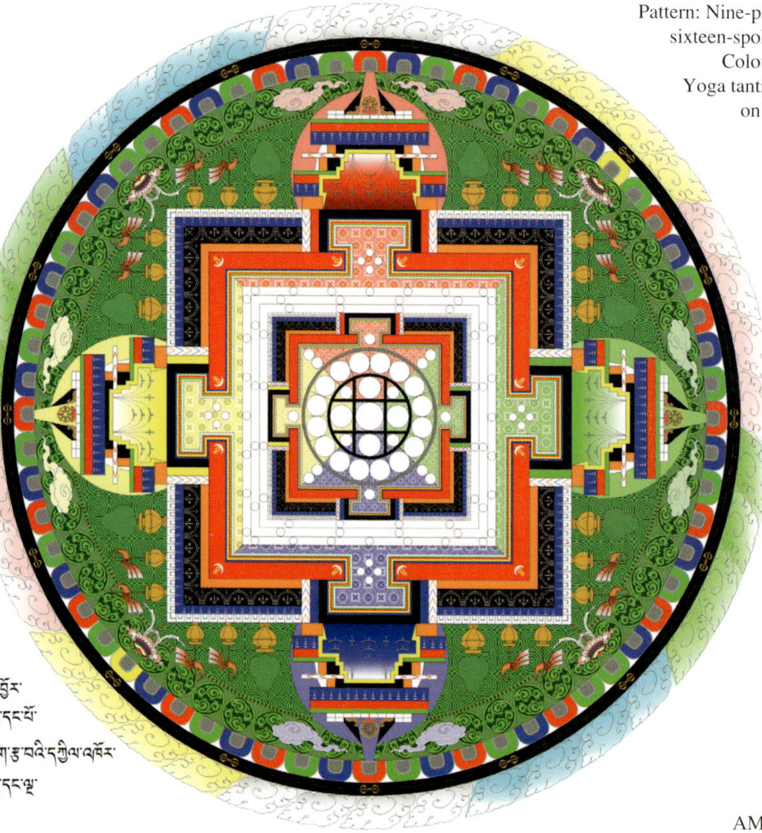

རྣལ་འབྱོར་
རྒྱུད་ཀྱི་དང་པོ་
ཀུན་རིག་རྩ་བའི་དཀྱིལ་འཁོར་
ལྷ་བརྒྱ་དང་ལྔ་

AMM: No. 12

The *Sarvadurgatipariśodhana-tantra* belonging to the Yoga tantras is one of the most popular tantras in Tibet since it was used for funerary rites. The Sarvavid-Vairocana-maṇḍala is the basic maṇḍala of this tantra, described first in the older of the two Tibetan translations of this text. It takes the form of a combination of a nine-panel grid and a sixteen-spoked wheel, and in the centre Sarvavid-Vairocana is depicted as the main deity. In the four cardinal directions around the main deity are Sarvadurgatipariśodhanarāja (east), Ratnaketu (south), Śākyakulendra (west) and Saṃkusumitarājendra (north). In the four intermediate directions of the central circle are Locanā (southeast), Māmakī (southwest), Pāṇḍarā (northwest) and Tārā (northeast). Between the sixteen spokes of the outside wheel are the sixteen great bodhisattvas of the Vajradhātu-maṇḍala (V-37). In the four intermediate directions outside the wheel are the four inner offering goddesses and the four outer offering goddesses, and in the four gates of the inner maṇḍala are the four gatekeepers Vajrāṅkuśa, Vajrapāśa, Vajrasphoṭa and Vajrāveśa. In the outer square are the sixteen bodhisattvas of the Auspicious Aeon (Bhadrakalpa), sixteen incomparable beings (*dpe bral gyi sems dpa'*), sixteen *śrāvaka*s and eight wrathful gatekeepers (accompanied by consorts). Thus, the total number of deities is 105. In addition, on the periphery of the outermost circle there should be Dharma-protecting deities, but these are omitted in the Hahn Foundation handscroll. It should be noted that there are several different opinions regarding the total number of deities in this maṇḍala, which is one of the most popular maṇḍalas in Tibet since it was frequently created for the benefit of a deceased person.

24. Thirteen-deity Aparimitāyus-maṇḍala

Pattern: 28b. Lotus + wheel;
Colour scheme:
Yoga tantras centred
on Amitābha

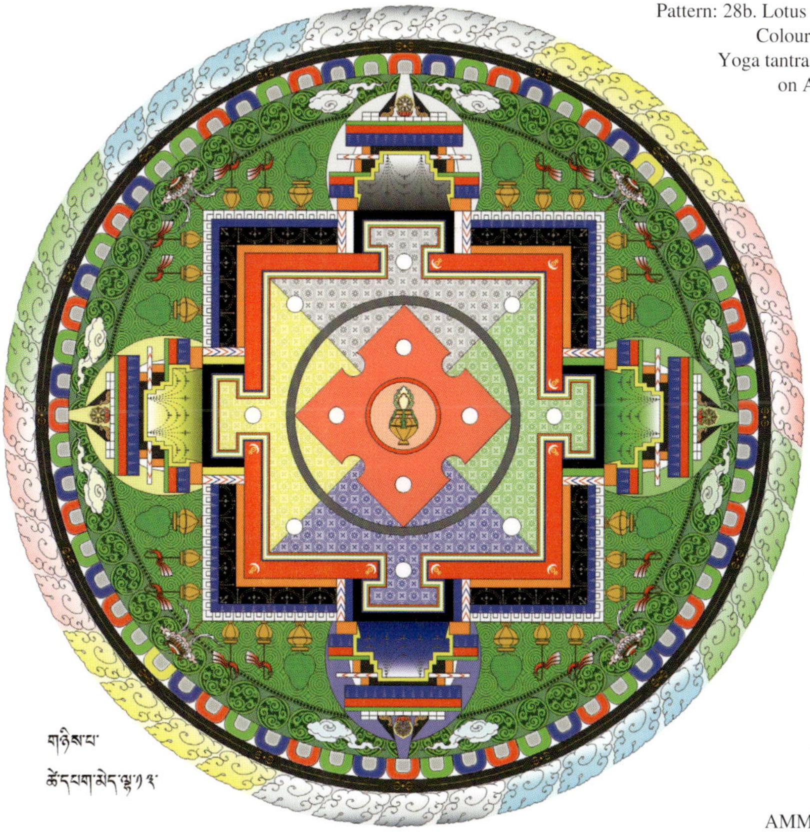

AMM: No. 17

The Aparimitāyus-maṇḍala is said to correspond to the fourth of the eleven or twelve maṇḍalas based on the *Sarvadurgatipariśodhana-tantra*, and it is called "Tshe dpag med gsuṅ," or "Aparimitāyus-Speech," because it is assigned to speech among the three mysteries of body, speech and mind. However, it is not explicitly described in the text of the tantra itself, and it is impossible to construct the maṇḍala without reference to commentaries and manuals. In the centre Aparimitāyus (here represented by a vase containing nectar) is depicted, and four Buddhas or four bodhisattvas are arranged in the four cardinal directions around the main deity. In the four intermediate directions outside the wheel are the four outer offering goddesses Vajradhūpā, Vajrapuṣpā, Vajradīpā and Vajragandhā, and in the four gates are the four female gatekeepers Aṅkuśī, Pāśī, Sphoṭā and Ghaṇṭā. Thus, this maṇḍala consists of thirteen deities. The colour scheme of the courtyard is that of the Yoga tantras centred on Amitābha (Type B), with the main deity having been changed from Vairocana to Amitābha. This is because Aparimitāyus is thought to be an emanation of Amitābha. *Roṅ tha's Iconometry* describes this maṇḍala as a combination of an eight-petalled lotus and a four-spoked wheel. However, many examples, including the Hahn Foundation handscroll, depict only a four-spoked wheel. Among the maṇḍalas described in the *Sarvadurgatipariśodhana-tantra*, examples of this maṇḍala are the most numerous after maṇḍalas of Sarvavid-Vairocana (M-23) and Navoṣṇīṣa (V-38). The Hahn Cultural Foundation possesses two other examples of coloured thangkas of this maṇḍala.

25. Thirteen-deity Vajrapāṇi-maṇḍala

Pattern: 28b. Lotus + wheel;
Colour scheme:
Highest Yoga tantras
centred on Akṣobhya

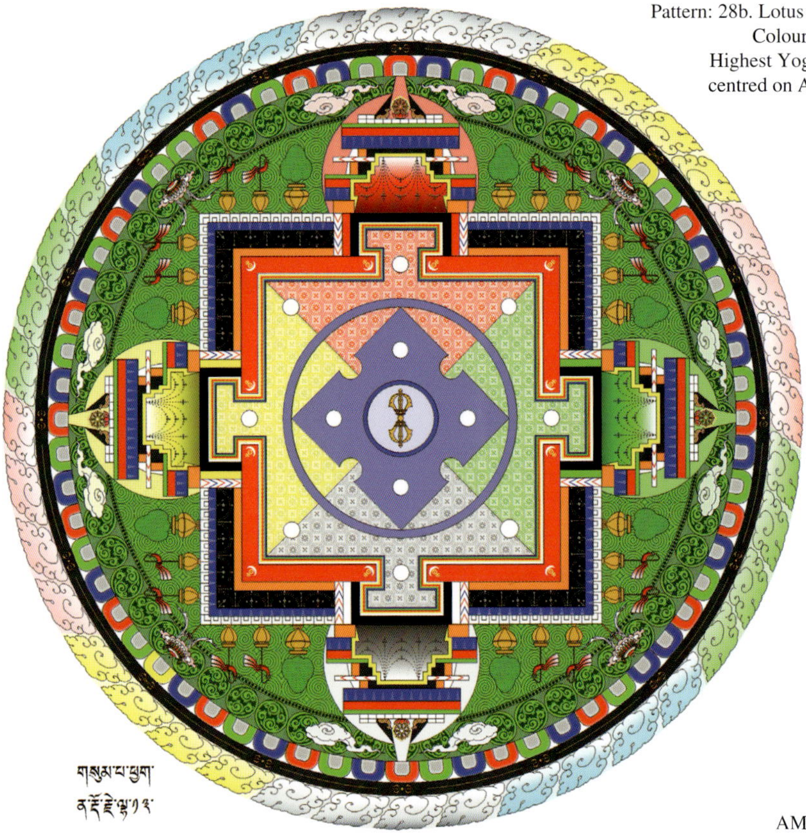

གསུམ་པ་ཕྱག
ན་རྡོ་རྗེ་ལྷ་༡༣་

AMM: No. 8

This maṇḍala is said to correspond to the third of the eleven or twelve maṇḍalas based on the *Sarvadurgatipariśodhana-tantra*, and it is called "Phyag na rdo rje thugs," or "Vajrapāṇi-Mind," because it is assigned to the mind among the three mysteries of body, speech and mind. In the centre Vajrapāṇi (here represented by a vajra) is depicted, and the four Buddhas Vairocana (east), Ratnasambhava (south), Amitābha (west) and Amoghasiddhi (north) are arranged in the four cardinal directions around the main deity. In the four intermediate directions outside the wheel are the four outer offering goddesses Vajradhūpā, Vajrapuṣpā, Vajradīpā and Vajragandhā, and in the four gates are the four gatekeepers Vajrāṅkuśa, Vajrapāśa, Vajrasphoṭa and Vajrāveśa. Thus, this maṇḍala consists of thirteen deities. Although it is classified among the Yoga tantras, the colour scheme of the courtyard is that of the Highest Yoga tantras centred on Akṣobhya (Type E) since it is centred on Vajrapāṇi, who belongs to the Vajra family presided over by Akṣobhya. *Roṅ tha's Iconometry* describes this maṇḍala, like the thirteen-deity Aparimitāyus-maṇḍala (M-24), as a combination of an eight-petalled lotus and a four-spoked wheel, but the Hahn Foundation handscroll depicts only a four-spoked wheel. Among the maṇḍalas described in the *Sarvadurgatipariśodhana-tantra*, examples of coloured thangkas depicting this maṇḍala, apart from maṇḍala sets, are rare.

26. One-hundred-and-thirty-eight-deity Vajrapāṇicakravartin-maṇḍala

Pattern: 30. Four-spoked wheel;
Colour scheme:
Highest Yoga tantras
centred on Akṣobhya

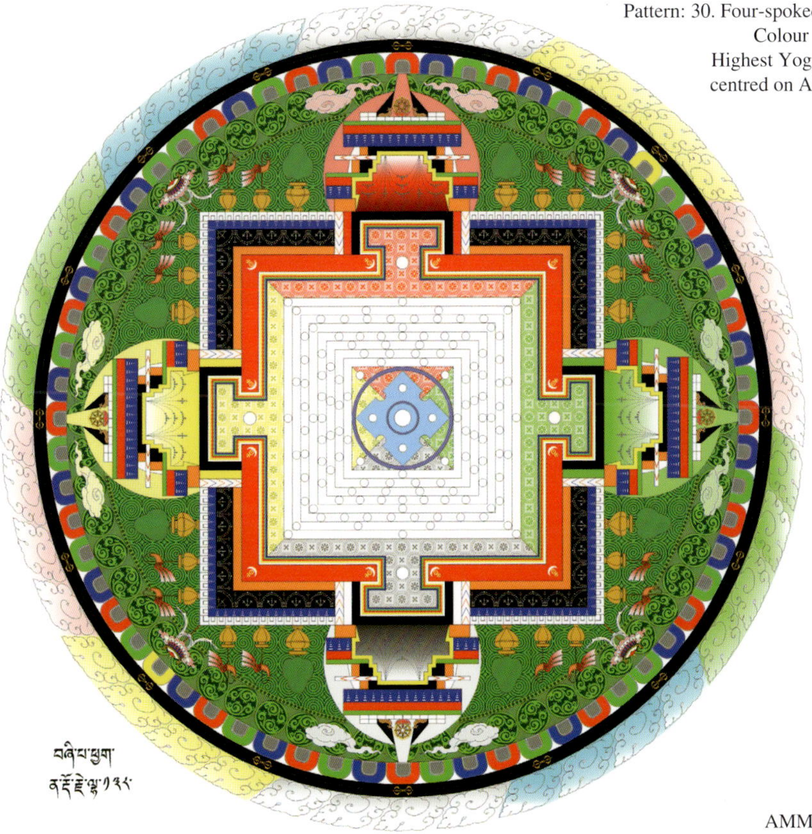

བཞི་པ་ཕྱག་
ན་རྡོ་རྗེ་ལྷ་༡༣༨

AMM: No. 18

This maṇḍala is the largest among the eleven or twelve maṇḍalas based on the *Sarvadurgatipariśodhana-tantra*, and it is said to correspond to the eleventh maṇḍala of this scripture. It is called "bDe ba chen po yon tan," or "Mahāsukha-Virtue," because it is assigned to virtue among the five categories of body, speech, mind, action and virtue. Vajrasattva is depicted on the hub of the four-spoked wheel, and four Buddhas or four Bodhisattvas are arranged in the four cardinal directions around the main deity. In the four corners of the inner square are the four Buddha-mothers, and in the eightfold outer square are the seven Buddhas of the past, the sixteen great bodhisattvas, the sixteen bodhisattvas of the Auspicious Aeon (Bhadrakalpa), sixteen *śrāvaka*s, twelve *pratyekabuddha*s, eight principal gods, eight planets, twenty-eight constellations, the four celestial kings and the protectors of the ten directions. In the four gates are the four gatekeepers Vajrāṅkuśa, Vajrapāśa, Vajrasphoṭa and Vajrāveśa. Thus, this maṇḍala consists of 138 deities. Although it is classified among the Yoga tantras, the colour scheme of the courtyard is that of the Highest Yoga tantras centred on Akṣobhya (Type E) since it is centred on Vajrasattva, who belongs to the Vajra family presided over by Akṣobhya. Among the maṇḍalas based on the *Sarvadurgatipariśodhana-tantra,* examples of this maṇḍala are relatively common. The Hahn Cultural Foundation and the Victoria and Albert Museum each possess a good example of a coloured thangka of this maṇḍala. However, both omit the four Buddha-mothers in the inner square, and the eightfold square has been replaced by eight concentric circles. Thus, there are slight differences in the arrangement of the deities and the iconometry.

27. Seventeen-deity Vajrajvālānalārka-maṇḍala

Pattern: 31. Twelve-spoked wheel;
Colour scheme:
Highest Yoga tantras
centred on Akṣobhya

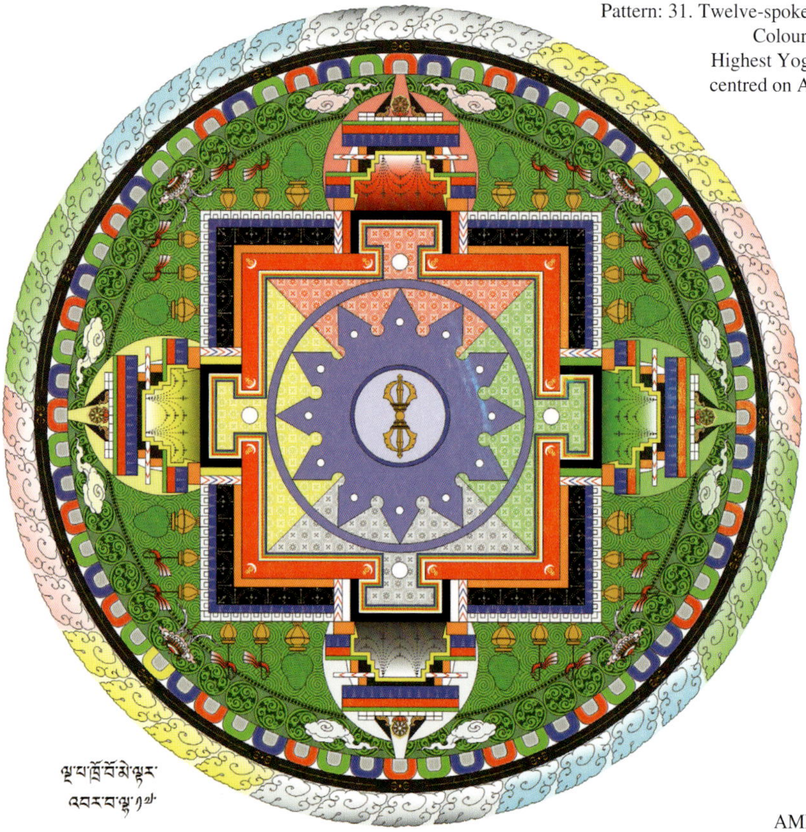

ལྷ་པ་ཁྲོ་བོ་མེ་ལྟར་
འབར་བ་ལྷ་༡༧

AMM: No. 9

This maṇḍala is said to correspond to the last of the eleven or twelve maṇḍalas based on the *Sarvadurgatipariśodhana-tantra*, and it is called "Me ltar 'bar ba phrin las," or "Jvālānalārka-Action," because it is assigned to action among the five categories of body, speech, mind, action and virtue. It takes the form of a twelve-spoked wheel, on the hub of which a wrathful deity named Vajrajvālānalārka (here represented by a vajra) is depicted as the main deity. On the twelve spokes are Trailokyavijaya, Loka gsum snaṅ (Sanskrit name unknown), Ṭakkirāja and Nīladaṇḍa (on the four central spokes), Amṛtakuṇḍalin, Hayagrīva, Mahābala and Acala (on the four spokes on the right), and Kālarākṣasī, Karmarākṣasī, Artharākṣasī and Upāyarākṣasī (on the four spokes on the left). In the four gates are the four female gatekeepers Kālāṅkuśī, Kālapāśī, Kālasphoṭā and Kālāveśā. The *Abhisamayamuktāmālā* and two commentaries on the *Sarvadurgatipariśodhana-tantra* by Vajravarman and Buddhaguhya differ somewhat with regard to the names and arrangement of the four *rākṣasī*s and four female gatekeepers. Although this maṇḍala is classified among the Yoga tantras, the colour scheme of the courtyard is that of the Highest Yoga tantras centred on Akṣobhya (Type E) since it is centred on Vajrajvālānalārka, who belongs to the Vajra family presided over by Akṣobhya. Among the maṇḍalas based on the *Sarvadurgatipariśodhana-tantra*, examples of coloured thangkas depicting this maṇḍala are rare, but one example is known to exist in a private collection in Japan.

28. Twenty-three-deity maṇḍala of Vajrapāṇi surrounded by the protectors of the ten directions and the four great kings

Pattern: 32. Lotus + wheel;
Colour scheme:
Highest Yoga tantras
centred on Akṣobhya

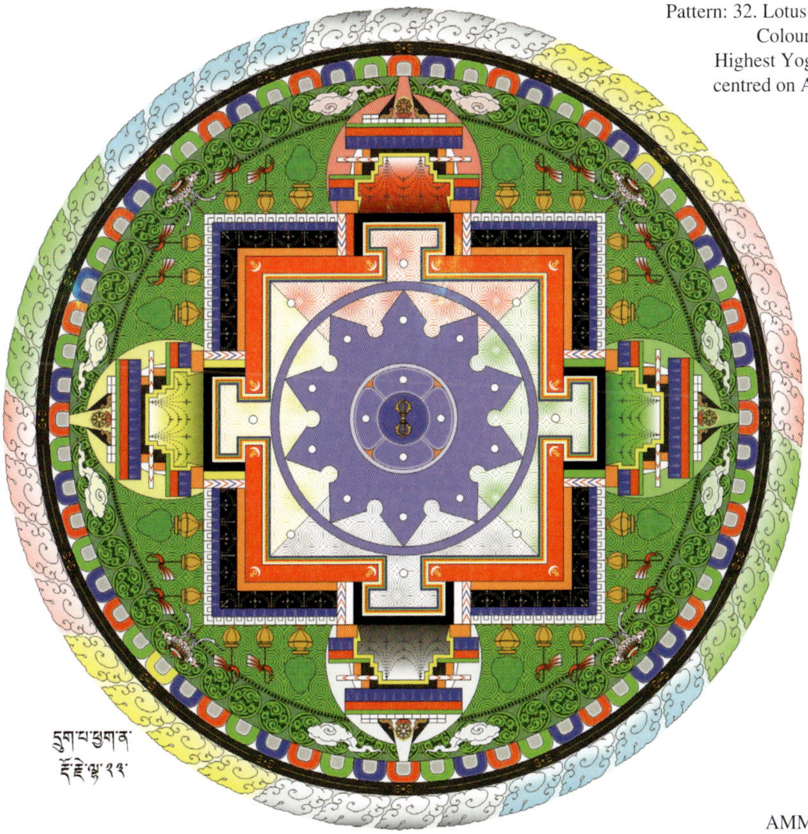

དྲུག་པ་ཕྱག་ན་
རྡོ་རྗེ་ལྷ་༢༣་

AMM: No. 62

This maṇḍala is thought to be a combination of "Vajrapāṇi surrounded by the four celestial kings" and "Vajrapāṇi surrounded by the protectors of the ten directions," the third and fourth of the eleven or twelve maṇḍalas based on the *Sarvadurgatipariśodhana-tantra*. It takes the form of a four-petalled lotus set on the hub of a ten-spoked wheel. On the pericarp of the lotus Vajrapāṇi (here represented by a vajra) is depicted, and on the four petals are the four celestial kings Dhṛtarāṣṭra (east), Virūḍhaka (south), Virūpākṣa (west) and Vaiśravaṇa (north). On the spokes of the outer wheel are the protectors of the ten directions, i.e., Indra (east), Agni (southeast), Yama (south), Nairṛti (southwest), Varuṇa (west), Vāyu (northwest), Vaiśravaṇa (north), Īśāna (northeast), Brahmā (top) and Pṛthivī (bottom). In the four corners are the four inner offering goddesses, and in the four gates are the four gatekeepers Vajrāṅkuśa, Vajrapāśa, Vajrasphoṭa and Vajrāveśa. Thus, the total number of deities is twenty-three. Although it is classified among the Yoga tantras, the colour scheme of the courtyard is that of the Highest Yoga tantras centred on Akṣobhya (Type E) since it is centred on Vajrapāṇi. The Ṅor maṇḍalas, meanwhile, include separately a maṇḍala of Vajrapāṇi surrounded by the four celestial kings (No. 33) and a maṇḍala of Vajrapāṇi surrounded by the protectors of the ten directions (No. 34). Both are frequently found in the sphere of Tibetan Buddhism, but the combining of these two maṇḍalas as in the present case is fairly rare.

29. Forty-five-deity Vajrapāṇi-maṇḍala

Pattern: 36c. Nine-panel grid + surrounding strips;
Colour scheme: Highest Yoga tantras centred on Akṣobhya

བདུན་པ་ཕྱག་ན་
རྡོ་རྗེ་ལྷ་༤༥་

AMM: No. 61

This maṇḍala is said to correspond to the sixth of the eleven or twelve maṇḍalas based on the *Sarvadurgatipariśodhana-tantra.* It is a maṇḍala depicting various deities symbolizing heavenly bodies and takes the form of a nine-panel grid surrounded by a square. In the centre, Vajrapāṇi (here represented by a vajra) is depicted as the main deity. In the eight directions surrounding the main deity are eight ascetics symbolizing eight planets, i.e., Moon (east), Sun (southeast), Saturn (south), Rāhu (southwest), Mars (west), Venus (northwest), Jupiter (north) and Mercury (northeast). Therefore, this maṇḍala is called "Draṅ sroṅ brgyad," or "Eight Ascetics." In the outer square are the twenty-eight constellations: Kṛttikā, Rohiṇī, Mṛgaśirā, Ārdrā, Punarvasu, Puṣya, Aśleṣā (east), Maghā, Pūrvaphalgunī, Uttaraphalgunī, Hastā, Citrā, Svātī, Viśākhā (south), Anurādhā, Jyeṣṭhā, Mūla, Pūrvāṣāḍhā, Uttarāṣāḍhā, Śravaṇā, Abhijit (west), Śatabhiṣā, Dhaniṣṭhā, Pūrvabhādrapadā, Uttarabhādrapadā, Revatī, Aśvinī and Bharaṇī (north). In addition, in the four corners are the four outer offering goddesses, and in the four gates are the four gatekeepers Vajrāṅkuśa, Vajrapāśa, Vajrasphoṭa and Vajrāveśa. Thus, the total number of deities is forty-five. Although it is classified among the Yoga tantras, the colour scheme of the courtyard is that of the Highest Yoga tantras centred on Akṣobhya (Type E) since it is centred on Vajrapāṇi. The Ṅor maṇḍalas include a maṇḍala of Trailokyavijaya surrounded by the *graha*s (planets) and *nakṣatra*s (constellations) (No. 35) which is centred on three-headed and four-armed Trailokyavijaya and, lacking the four outer offering goddesses, consists of forty-one deities.

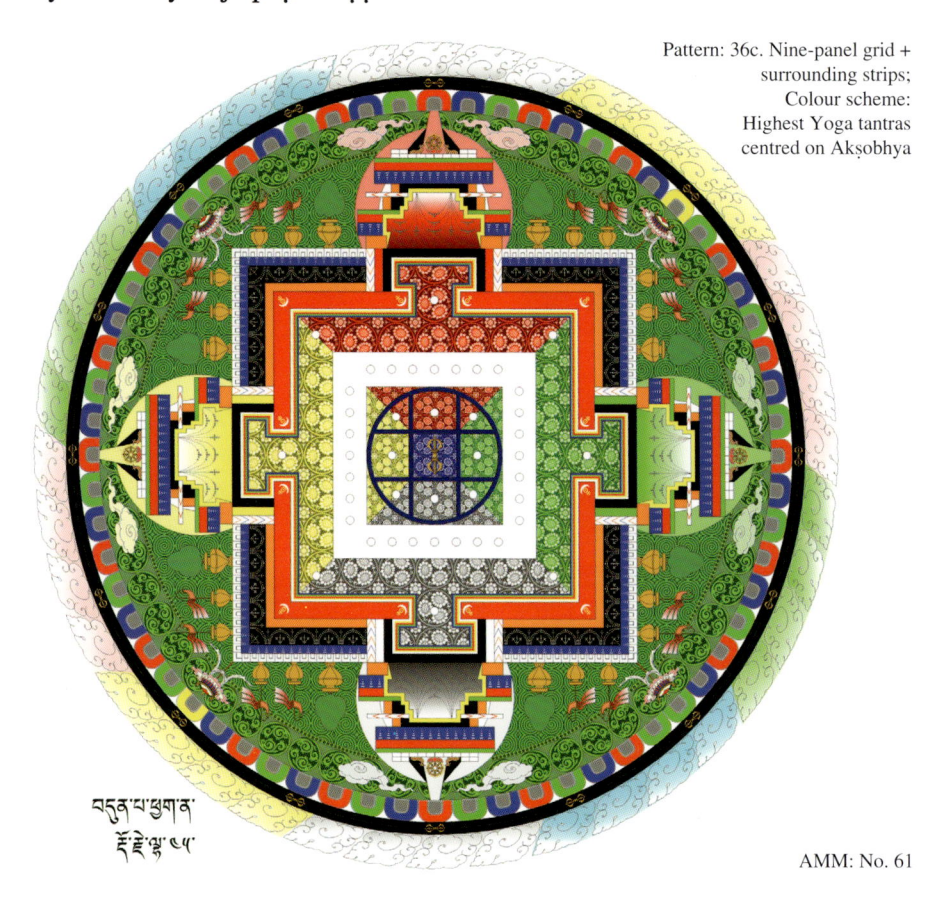

30. Thirteen-deity maṇḍala of Vajrapāṇi surrounded by the eight great *nāga*s

Pattern: 29. Eight-petalled lotus;
Colour scheme:
Highest Yoga tantras
centred on Akṣobhya

AMM: No. 63

This maṇḍala corresponds to the seventh of the eleven or twelve maṇḍalas based on the *Sarvadurgatipariśodhana-tantra.* It takes the form of an eight-petalled lotus, on the pericarp of which Vajrapāṇi (here represented by a vajra) is depicted. On the eight lotus petals are the eight great *nāga*s, i.e., Ananta (east), Takṣaka (south), Karkoṭaka (west), Kulika (north), Vāsuki (southeast), Śaṅkhapāla (southwest), Padma (northwest) and Varuṇa (northeast). When compared with other maṇḍalas, the central eight-petalled lotus is quite small. *Roṅ tha's Iconometry* stipulates that one should depict an eight-petalled lotus inside the outer square. The *Abhisamayamuktāmālā*, only explaining that one should visualize the four families as gatekeepers, does not give the names of the four gatekeepers. 'On rgyal sras explains this as a reference to the four castes, starting with *kṣatriya*s. The Ṅor maṇḍalas include a maṇḍala of Vajrapāṇi surrounded by the eight great *nāga*s (No. 36), and it lacks the four gatekeepers. The *rGyud sde kun btus* (Collection of All Tantras) interprets them as the four gatekeepers starting with Vajrāṅkuśa. Although it is classified among the Yoga tantras, the colour scheme of the courtyard is that of the Highest Yoga tantras centred on Akṣobhya (Type E) since it is centred on Vajrapāṇi.

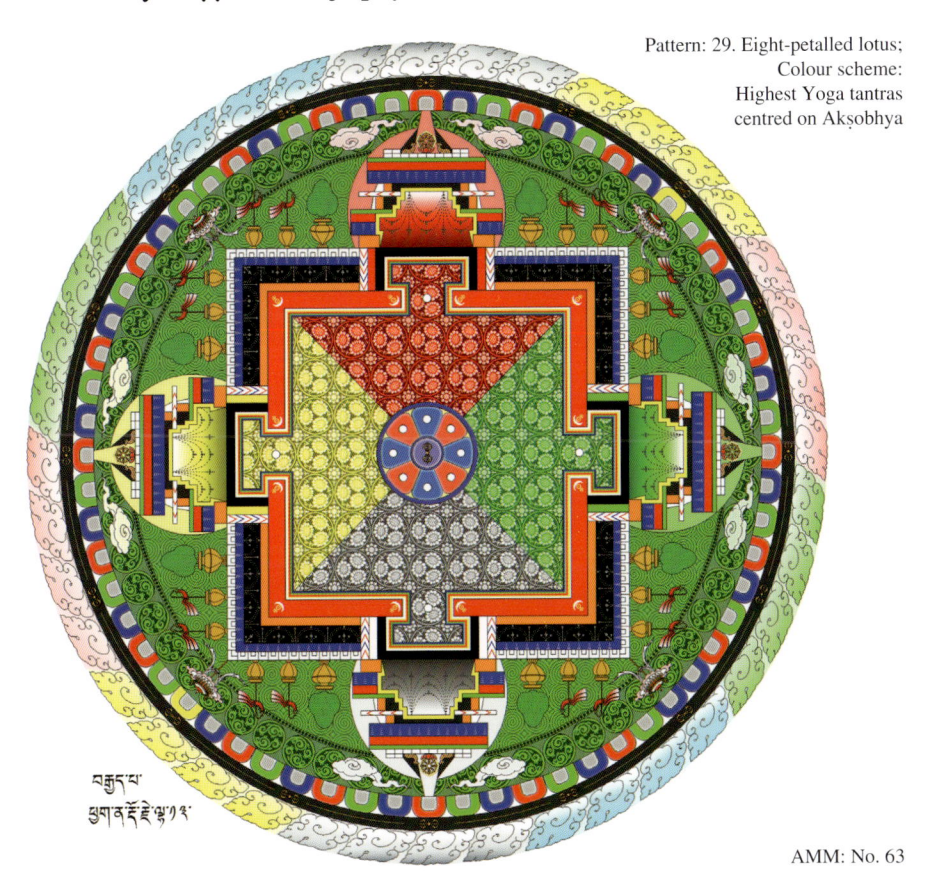

31. Fifty-seven-deity Trailokyavijaya-maṇḍala

Pattern: 25. Eight-petalled lotus + nine-panel grid;
Colour scheme: Highest Yoga tantras centred on Akṣobhya

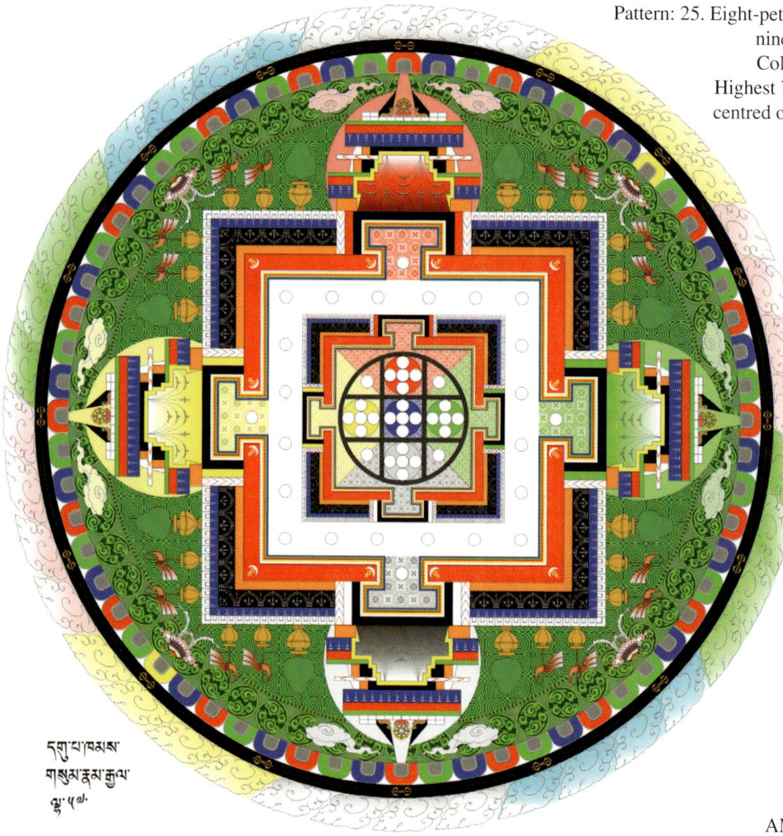

AMM: No. 16

This maṇḍala is the basic maṇḍala of Chapter II of the *Sarvatathāgatatattvasaṃgraha,* the root text of the Yoga tantras, and corresponds to the Gōzanze-e (Trailokyavijaya-maṇḍala) of the Sino-Japanese Vajradhātu-maṇḍala, which consists of nine maṇḍalas. It consists of fifty-three deities: five Buddhas, four *pāramitā* goddesses, sixteen great bodhisattvas, eight offering goddesses, four gatekeepers and the sixteen bodhisattvas of the Auspicious Aeon (Bhadrakalpa). The Hahn Foundation handscroll depicts a double pavilion, and the four gatekeepers are also duplicated. The inscription of the Hahn Foundation handscroll gives the total number of deities as fifty-seven (although it does not depict the four gatekeepers of the inner maṇḍala). According to *Roṅ tha's Iconometry*, this maṇḍala takes the form of four-petalled lotuses set in a nine-panel grid as in the Vajradhātu-maṇḍala (V-37). However, the Hahn Foundation handscroll depicts five lunar discs set in a nine-panel grid, like the Sino-Japanese Vajradhātu-maṇḍala. Moreover, the Hahn Foundation handscroll depicts the four outer offering goddesses, four gatekeepers and sixteen bodhisattvas of the Auspicious Aeon in the outer maṇḍala and omits the twenty protective deities of the Outer Vajra family which are explained in Chapter II of the *Sarvatathāgatatattva-saṃgraha.* The colour scheme of the courtyard ought to be that of the Yoga tantras centred on Vairocana since this maṇḍala is centred on Vairocana even though it is classified as belonging to the Vajra family. However, the Hahn Foundation handscroll adopts an unusual colour scheme, that of the Highest Yoga tantras centred on Akṣobhya, since Mitrayogin changed the main deity from Vairocana to Trailokyavijaya in his *Abhisamayamuktāmālā*.

32. Fifty-seven-deity Sarvārthasiddhi-maṇḍala

Pattern: 25. Eight-petalled lotus + nine-panel grid;
Colour scheme: Yoga tantras centred on Vairocana

བཅུ་པ་དོན་
ཀུན་གྲུབ་པ་ལྷ་༥༧་

AMM: No. 14

This maṇḍala is the basic maṇḍala of Chapter IV of the *Sarvatathāgatatattvasaṃgraha,* and all of the deities except the five Buddhas are emanations of Ākāśagarbha. Like the Trailokyavijaya-maṇḍala (M-31), this maṇḍala consists of five Buddhas, sixteen great bodhisattvas, four *pāramitā* goddesses, eight offering goddesses, four gatekeepers and the sixteen bodhisattvas of the Auspicious Aeon (Bhadrakalpa). Thus, this maṇḍala consists of fifty-three deities since it does not have a double pavilion and has no need to duplicate the gatekeepers as in the Trailokyavijaya-maṇḍala (M-31). Therefore, the inscription of the Hahn Foundation handscroll would seem to be in error when it gives the total number of deities as fifty-seven. According to *Roṅ tha's Iconometry*, this maṇḍala takes the form of nine four-petalled lotuses set in a nine-panel grid as in the Vajradhātu-maṇḍala (V-37). However, the Hahn Foundation handscroll depicts only a four-petalled lotus set in the central panel, where Vairocana and the four *pāramitā* goddesses are depicted. Although it is classified as belonging to the Jewel family represented by Ākāśagarbha, the colour scheme of the courtyard is that of the Yoga tantras centred on Vairocana (Type A) since it is centred on Vairocana. The Sarvārthasiddhi-maṇḍala is not included in any other maṇḍala sets, and a wall painting (15th century) in the north chapel in the dome (*bum pa*) of the Great Stūpa of dPal 'khor chos sde in rGyal rtse may be the only extant example of this maṇḍala.

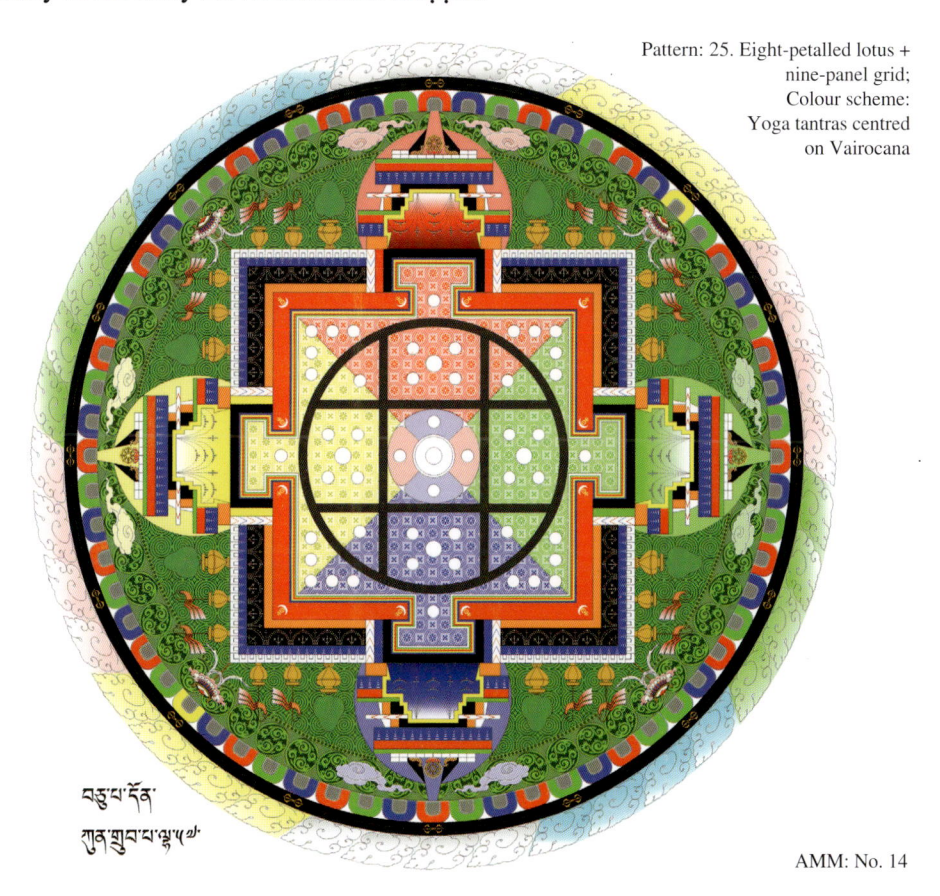

33. Fifty-seven-deity Sarvajagadvinaya-maṇḍala

Pattern: 25. Eight-petalled lotus + nine-panel grid;
Colour scheme: Yoga tantras centred on Vairocana

བཅུ་གཅིག་པ་
འགྲོ་བ་འདུལ་བ་
ལྷ་ ༥༧་

AMM: No. 15

This maṇḍala is the basic maṇḍala of Chapter III of the *Sarvatathāgatatattvasaṃgraha,* and all of the deities except the five Buddhas, such as Ekādaśamukha, Hayagrīva and Amoghapāśa, are emanations of Avalokiteśvara. Like the Trailokyavijaya-maṇḍala (M-31), this maṇḍala consists of five Buddhas, sixteen great bodhisattvas, four *pāramitā* goddesses, eight offering goddesses, four gatekeepers and the sixteen bodhisattvas of the Auspicious Aeon (Bhadrakalpa). Thus, this maṇḍala consists of fifty-three deities. Like the Sarvārthasiddhi-maṇḍala (M-32), it does not have a double pavilion and has no need to duplicate the gatekeepers. Therefore, the inscription of the Hahn Foundation handscroll would seem to be in error when it gives the total number of deities as fifty-seven. According to *Roṅ tha's Iconometry*, it takes the form of nine four-petalled lotuses set in a nine-panel grid as in the Vajradhātu-maṇḍala (V-37). However, the Hahn Foundation handscroll depicts it as a square nine-panel grid rotated at an angle of forty-five degrees. This pattern also appears in the only extant example of this maṇḍala in the dome (*bum pa*) of the Great Stūpa of dPal 'khor chos sde in rGyal rtse. This fact shows that the editor of the Hahn Foundation handscroll was versed in the iconography of Esoteric Buddhism. Although it is classified as belonging to the Lotus family represented by Avalokiteśvara, the colour scheme of the courtyard is that of the Yoga tantras centred on Vairocana (Type A) since it is centred on Vairocana.

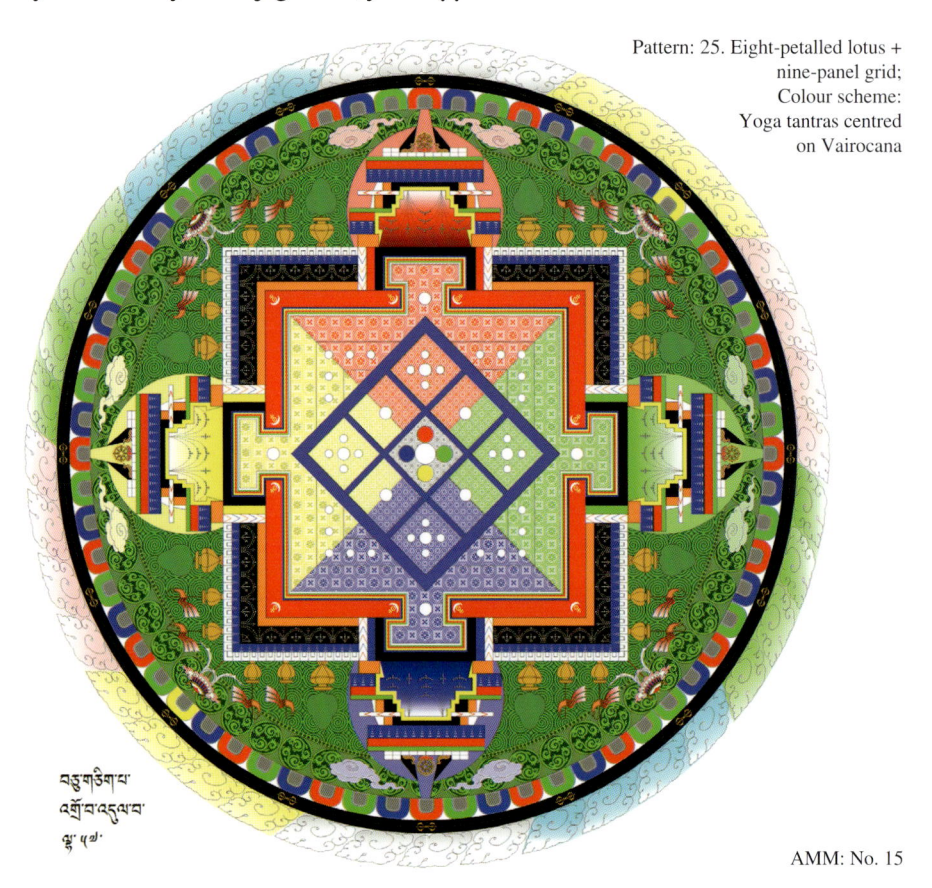

34. Sixty-one-deity Paramādya-Vajrasattva-maṇḍala

Pattern: 25. Eight-petalled lotus + nine-panel grid;
Colour scheme: *Paramādya-tantra*

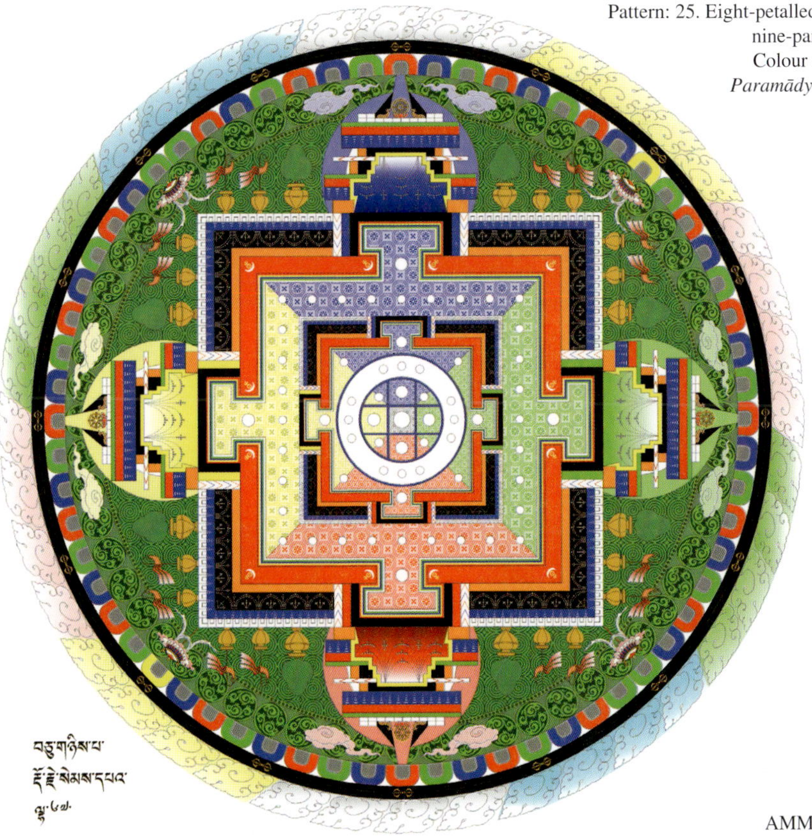

AMM: No. 11

The *Paramādya-tantra* is a development of the *Prajñāpāramitānaya-sūtra*, and in Tibet it is classified among the Yoga tantras like the *Sarvatathāgatatattvasaṃgraha*. It describes many maṇḍalas, among which the Vajrasattva-maṇḍala is the first, being explained at the beginning of this scripture. The inner pavilion takes the form of a nine-panel grid, in the centre of which Vajrasattva is depicted as the main deity. Vajramanodbhava (east), Kelikīla (south), Vajranismara (west) and Vajragarva (north) are arranged in the four cardinal directions around the main deity, and in the four intermediate directions of the central circle are the offering goddesses of the four seasons, i.e., Vajrarati (southeast), Mahāratavajrī (southwest), Vajralocanī (northwest) and Mahāśrī (northeast). They are the same as the attendant deities of the Rishu-e (maṇḍala of the *Prajñāpāramitānaya-sūtra*) in the Sino-Japanese Vajradhātu-maṇḍala, which consists of nine maṇḍalas. In the four cardinal directions are the four Buddhas Akṣobhya (east), Ratnasambhava (south), Amitābha (west) and Amoghasiddhi (north), who are each accompanied by two of the eight great bodhisattvas of the *Prajñāpāramitānaya-sūtra.* In the four gates of the inner and outer pavilions are the four gatekeepers Rūpā, Śabdā, Gandhā and Rasā (eight in total), in the four corners of the outer pavilion are the four goddesses Lāsyā, Hāsyā, Gītā and Nṛtyā, and in each of the four strips of the outer pavilion are seven protective deities. Thus, the total number of deities is sixty-one. This maṇḍala adopts an unusual colour scheme consisting of red (east), yellow (south), blue (west) and green (north).

35. Fifty-three-deity Mañjughoṣa-maṇḍala (as transmitted by Vilāsavajra)

Pattern: 25. Eight-petalled lotus + nine-panel grid;
Colour scheme: Yoga tantras centred on Vairocana

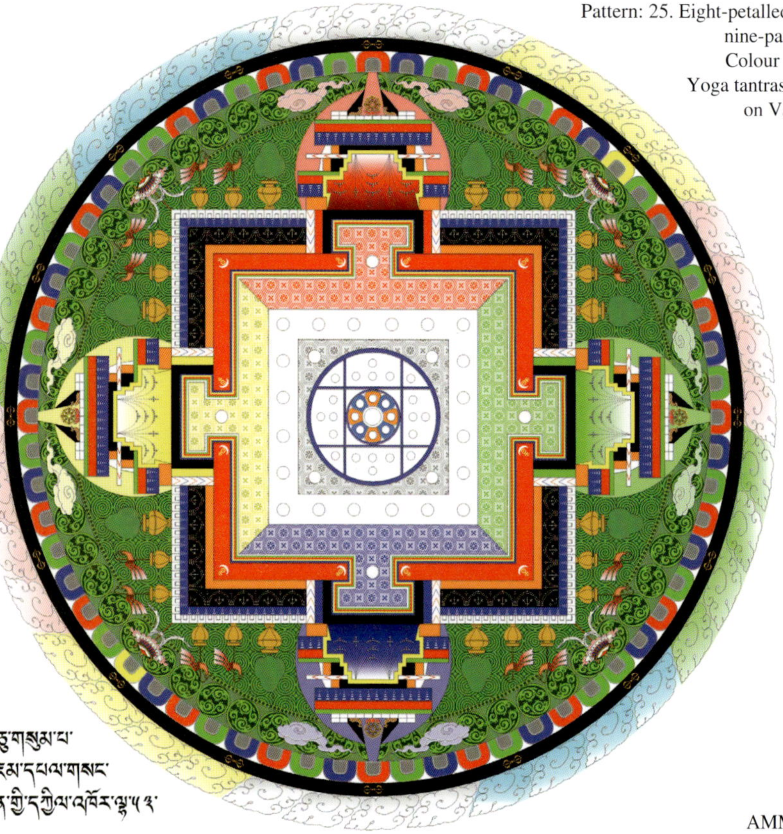

བཅུ་གསུམ་པ་
འཇམ་དཔལ་གསང་
ལྡན་གྱི་དཀྱིལ་འཁོར་ལྷ་༥༣་

AMM: No. 4

This maṇḍala belongs to the school of Vilāsavajra (8th century), called *gSaṅ ldan* in Tibet, which was a school of interpretation of the *Mañjuśrīnāmasaṅgīti*. In Tibet, images based on this tradition have been produced until recently. This maṇḍala takes the form of an eight-petalled lotus set in the centre of a nine-panel grid surrounded by a square. On the pericarp of the lotus Mañjughoṣa-jñānasattva is depicted as the main deity. On the lotus petals in the four cardinal directions there are depicted four kinds of Mañjuśrī, i.e., Vajrakhaḍga (east), Prajñājñāna (south), Arapacana (west) and Jñānakāya (north), and on the lotus petals in the four intermediate directions are the four *pāramitā*s. In each of the panels in the four cardinal directions are four of the sixteen great bodhisattvas; in the panels in the intermediate directions are the four inner offering goddesses Lāsyā, Mālā, Gītā and Nṛtyā; in the four strips of the outer square are the sixteen bodhisattvas of the Auspicious Aeon (Bhadrakalpa) and the four outer offering goddesses; and in the four gates are the four gatekeepers starting with Vajrāṅkuśa. Thus, this maṇḍala consists of fifty-three deities. The Hahn Foundation handscroll depicts fifty-seven seats for the deities in this maṇḍala even though the inscription gives the total number of deities as fifty-three. This may be due to a mistaken duplication of four offering goddesses. The colour scheme of the courtyard is that of the Yoga tantras centred on Vairocana (Type A) since it is centred on Mañjughoṣa-jñānasattva, who belongs to the Tathāgata family presided over by Vairocana.

36. Seventeen-deity Mañjughoṣa-maṇḍala (as transmitted by Candragomin)

Pattern: 26. Nine-panel grid;
Colour scheme:
Yoga tantras centred
on Vairocana

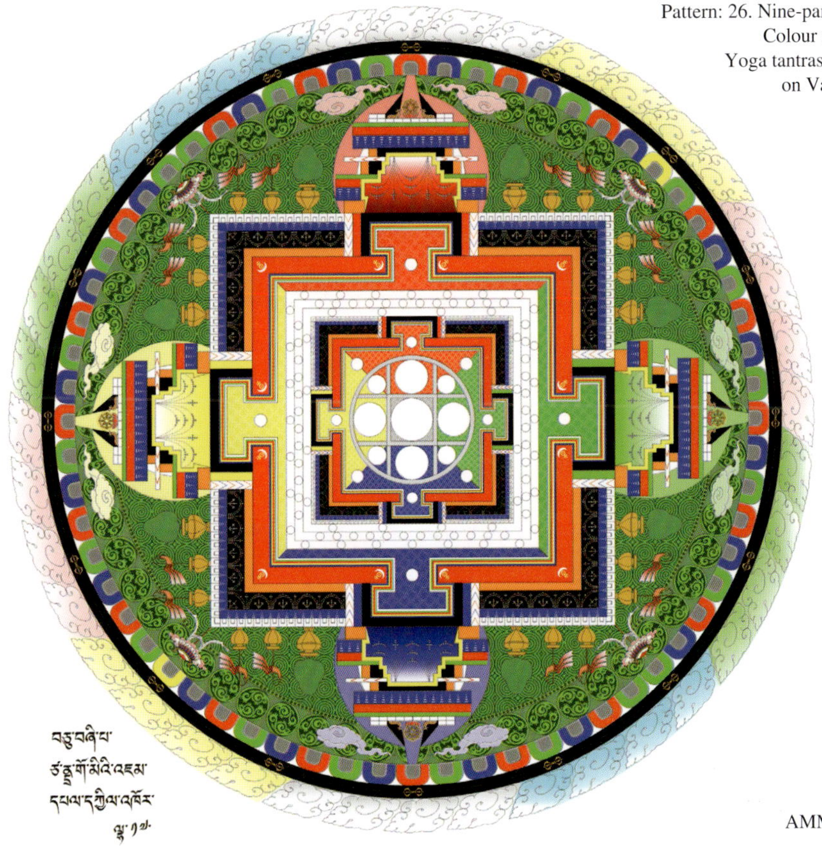

བཅུ་བཞི་པ་
ཙནྡྲ་གོ་མིའི་འཇམ་
དཔལ་དཀྱིལ་འཁོར་

AMM: No. 5

Candragomin was an Indian Buddhist scholar who composed a Sanskrit grammar and an extensive commentary on the *Mañjuśrīnāmasaṅgīti* (Peking No. 3363). *A History of Tibetan Buddhism* records that he engaged in debate with the Mādhyamika philosopher Candrakīrti, but this is improbable since, according to modern research, he was active in the first half of the tenth century. This maṇḍala is based on his interpretation of the *Mañjuśrīnāmasaṅgīti.* The centre of the inner pavilion takes the form of a nine-panel grid, in the centre of which Mañjughoṣa-jñānasattva is depicted as the main deity. Akṣobhya (east), Ratnasambhava (south), Amitābha (west) and Amoghasiddhi (north) are arranged in the four cardinal directions around the main deity, and in the four intermediate directions are the four Buddha-mothers. In the four corners are the four inner offering goddesses, and in the four gates are the four gatekeepers starting with Vajrāṅkuśa. Thus, the number of deities in the inner pavilion is seventeen. The outer pavilion takes the form of a triple square, and in the first square are the sixteen bodhisattvas of the Auspicious Aeon (Bhadrakalpa), in the second square goddesses who are deifications of doctrinal categories of Buddhism, and in the third square twenty-eight constellations. The four gates are occupied by the four celestial kings. Thus, the total number of deities is 133. However, the inscription of the Hahn Foundation handscroll does not count the deities in the outer pavilion. The colour scheme of the courtyard is that of the Yoga tantras centred on Vairocana (Type A) since it is centred on Mañjughoṣa-jñānasattva, who belongs to the Tathāgata family presided over by Vairocana.

37. Twenty-one-deity Mañjughoṣa-maṇḍala (profound tradition)

Pattern: 27. Four-petalled lotus + sixteen-spoked wheel;
Colour scheme: Yoga tantras centred on Vairocana

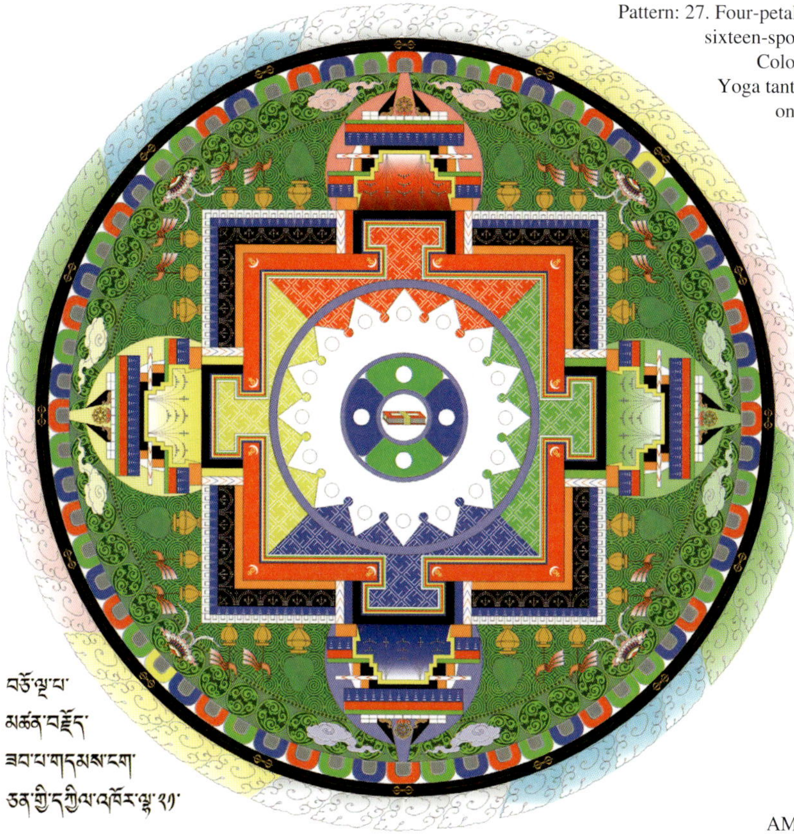

བཅོ་ལྔ་པ་
མཚན་བརྗོད་
ཟབ་པ་གདམས་ངག་
ཅན་གྱི་དཀྱིལ་འཁོར་ལྷ་༢༡་

AMM: No. 76

This maṇḍala is also based on the *Mañjuśrīnāmasaṅgīti* and is centred on Mañjughoṣa-jñānasattva. It takes the form of a four-petalled lotus set on the hub of a sixteen-spoked wheel. On the pericarp of the four-petalled-lotus Mañjughoṣa-jñānasattva (here represented by a manuscript of the *Prajñāpāramitā-sūtra*) is depicted as the main deity, and on the lotus petals in the four cardinal directions the four *pāramitā*s—Sattvavajrī (east), Ratnavajrī (south), Dharmavajrī (west) and Karmavajrī (north)—are arranged around the main deity. On the sixteen spokes of the outer wheel are the sixteen great bodhisattvas of the Vajradhātu-maṇḍala: Vajrasattva, Vajrarāja, Vajrarāga and Vajrasādhu (east), Vajraratna, Vajrateja, Vajraketu and Vajrahāsa (south), Vajradharma, Vajratīkṣṇa, Vajrahetu and Vajrabhāṣa (west), and Vajrakarma, Vajrarakṣa, Vajrayakṣa and Vajrasandhi (north). The colour scheme of the courtyard is that of the Yoga tantras centred on Vairocana (Type A) since it is centred on Mañjughoṣa-jñānasattva, who belongs to the Tathāgata family presided over by Vairocana. In Tibet, the *Mañjuśrīnāmasaṅgīti* is very popular as a text used for daily recitaton. There are also many examples of the Dharmadhātuvāgīśvara-maṇḍala (V-39) based on this text, and maṇḍalas of the Vilāsavajra tradition (cf. M-35) were also produced. However, this maṇḍala is not included in any other maṇḍala sets, nor has any coloured thangka depicting this maṇḍala been identified.

38. Sixty-four-deity Prajñāpāramitā-maṇḍala

Pattern: 35. Eight petalled lotus + ten four-petalled lotuses; Colour scheme: Highest Yoga tantras centred on Akṣobhya

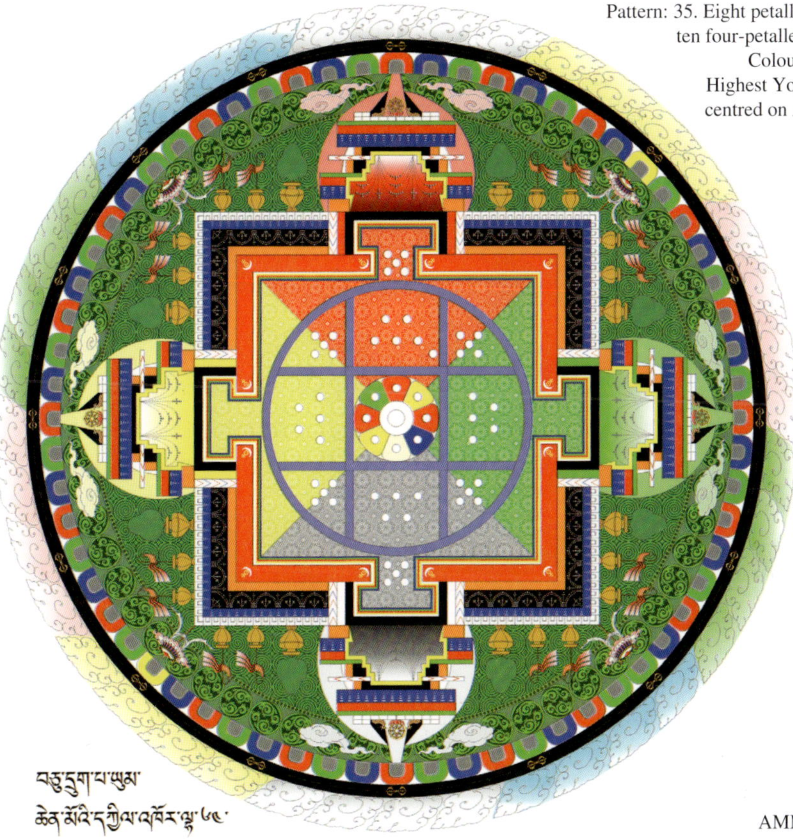

བཅུ་དྲུག་པ་ཡུམ་
ཆེན་མོའི་དཀྱིལ་འཁོར་ལྷ་༦༤་

AMM: No. 72

Prajñāpāramitā is a deification of the *Prajñāpāramitā-sūtra*, the root scripture of Mahāyāna Buddhism. She is depicted as a beautiful goddess since *prajñāpāramitā* is a feminine noun, and in Tibet she was called "Yum chen mo," or "Great Mother." This maṇḍala takes the form of an eight-petalled lotus in the centre of a nine-panel grid, and Prajñāpāramitā is depicted on the pericarp of the lotus. On the eight petals surrounding the main deity are the four Buddha-mothers and four *pāramitā* goddesses. In the four cardinal directions and four intermediate directions and at the top and bottom of the nine-panel grid the Buddhas of the ten directions, each accompanied by four bodhisattvas, are depicted. *Roṅ tha's Iconometry* explains that there should be an eight-petalled lotus in the centre of the nine-panel grid and ten four-petalled lotuses in the four cardinal directions and four intermediate directions and at the top and bottom, but the Hahn Foundation handscroll omits all the lotuses except an eight-petalled lotus in the centre. In Tibet and Nepal, Prajñāpāramitā is widely worshipped, and many images of Prajñāpāramitā can be seen, but examples of maṇḍalas of Prajñāpāramitā are rare. There are three maṇḍalas centred on Prajñāpāramitā (15th century) in the north chapel in the dome (*bum pa*) of the Great Stūpa of dPal 'khor chos sde in rGyal rtse, but none of them are identical with this maṇḍala.

39. One-hundred-deity maṇḍala of the one hundred clans

Pattern: 33. Eight petalled lotus + eight-spoked wheel;
Colour scheme: Highest Yoga tantras centred on Akṣobhya

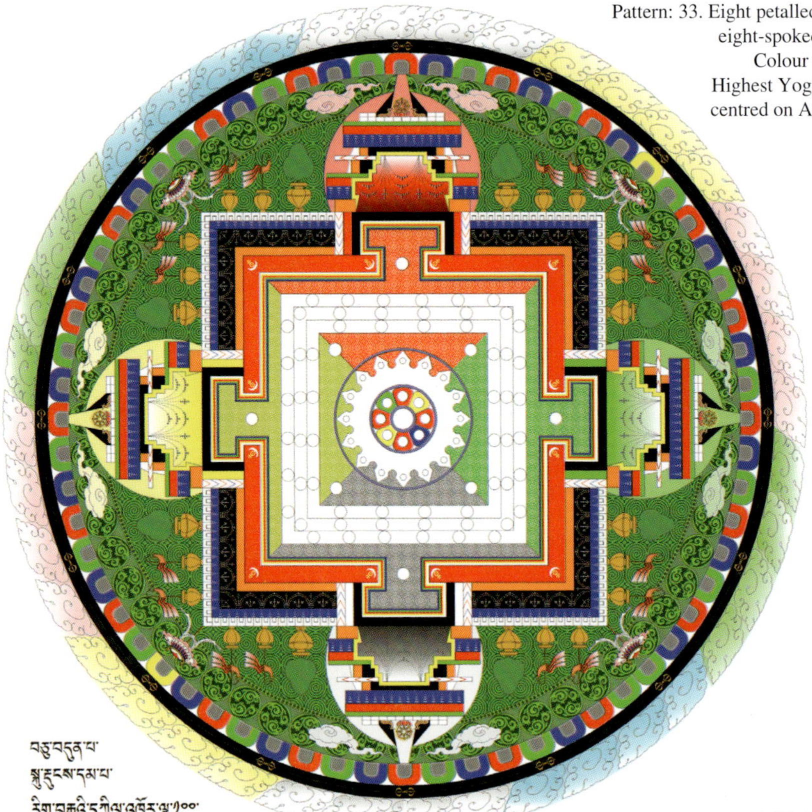

བཅུ་བདུན་པ་
སྐྱུ་རྡུངས་དམ་པ་
རིག་བརྒྱའི་དཀྱིལ་འཁོར་ལྷ་༡༠༠་

AMM: No. 100

The "one hundred clans" represent the idea that the five families, the basis of the Vajradhātu-maṇḍala and the Yoga tantras, further evolved into one hundred clans through their mutual interpenetration, and this maṇḍala symbolizes this idea in the form of a maṇḍala consisting of one hundred deities. It takes the form of a combination of an eight-petalled lotus and a sixteen-spoked wheel (or an eight-spoked wheel according to *Roṅ tha's Iconometry*) surrounded by a triple square, and on the pericarp of the lotus Sarvavid-Vairocana is depicted as the main deity. In the four cardinal directions around the main deity are Sarvadurgatipariśodhanarāja (east), Ratnaketu (south), Śākyakulendra (west) and Saṃkusumitarājendra (north). In the four intermediate directions of the central circle are Locanā (southeast), Māmakī (southwest), Pāṇḍarā (northwest) and Tārā (northeast). On the sixteen spokes of the outer wheel are the sixteen great bodhisattvas of the Vajradhātu-maṇḍala, and in the four intermediate directions outside the wheel are the four inner offering goddesses. In the first outer square are the sixteen bodhisattvas of the Auspicious Aeon (Bhadrakalpa), in the second square are sixteen incomparable beings (*dpe bral gyi sems dpa'*) and the four outer offering goddesses, and in the third square are sixteen *śrāvaka*s and twelve *pratyekabuddha*s. In the four gates are the four gatekeepers starting with Vajrāṅkuśa and the four celestial kings. Thus, the total number of deities is 101. In this way, this maṇḍala was structured with reference to the Sarvavid-Vairocana-maṇḍala (M-23) as a maṇḍala consisting of the one hundred clans. The inscription of the Hahn Foundation handscroll gives the number of deities as one hundred, but only ninety-seven seats for deities are depicted. The colour scheme of the courtyard ought to be that of the Yoga tantras centred on Vairocana, but for some unknown reason the Hahn Foundation handscroll has adopted the colour scheme of the Highest Yoga tantras centred on Akṣobhya.

40. Seventeen-deity Vajrasattva-maṇḍala

Pattern: 34. Eight-spoked wheel;
Colour scheme:
Highest Yoga tantras
centred on Akṣobhya

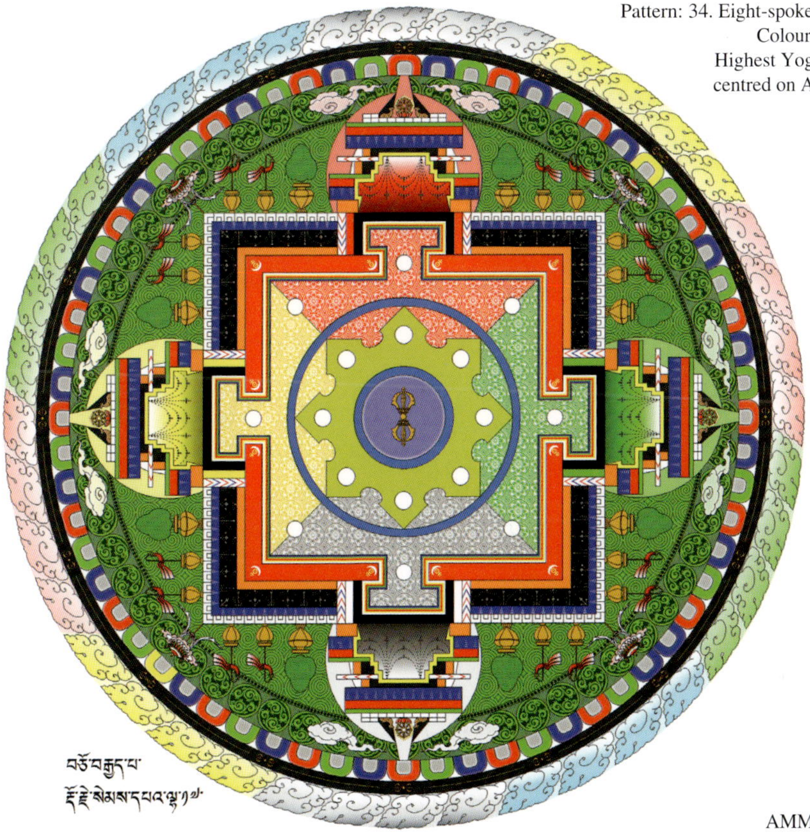

བཅོ་བརྒྱད་པ་
རྡོ་རྗེ་སེམས་དཔའ་ལྷ་༡༧་

AMM: No. 78

According to the *Abhisamayamuktāmālā*, this maṇḍala is centred on Vajrasattva, who has a mantra of one hundred syllables (*śatākṣara*). This mantra is expounded in many Esoteric Buddhist scriptures, starting with the *Sarvatathāgatatattvasaṃgraha*, and is thought to be effective for purifying the sin of breaking a pledge and for protecting a practitioner. This maṇḍala takes the form of an eight-spoked wheel, on the hub of which is Vajrasattva (here represented by a vajra), who holds a vajra in his right hand and draws a bell towards his body with his left hand. On the spokes in the four cardinal directions around the main deity are Vairocana (east), Ratnasambhava (south), Amitābha (west) and Amoghasiddhi (north). On the spokes in the four intermediate directions are the four Buddha-mothers Locanā (southeast), Māmakī (southwest), Pāṇḍarā (northwest) and Tārā (northeast). In the four corners are the four outer offering goddesses, and in the four gates are the four gatekeepers starting with Vajrāṅkuśa. Thus, the total number of deities is seventeeen. Although it is classified among the Yoga tantras, the colour scheme of the courtyard is that of the Highest Yoga tantras centred on Akṣobhya (Type E) since it is centred on Vajrasattva. According to 'On rgyal sras, the Buddha in the east is Akṣobhya, but it ought to be Vairocana if the colour scheme centred on Akṣobhya is adopted.

41. Twenty-one-deity maṇḍala of six-headed Yamāntaka

Pattern: 12. Eight-spoked wheel;
Colour scheme:
Highest Yoga tantras
centred on Akṣobhya

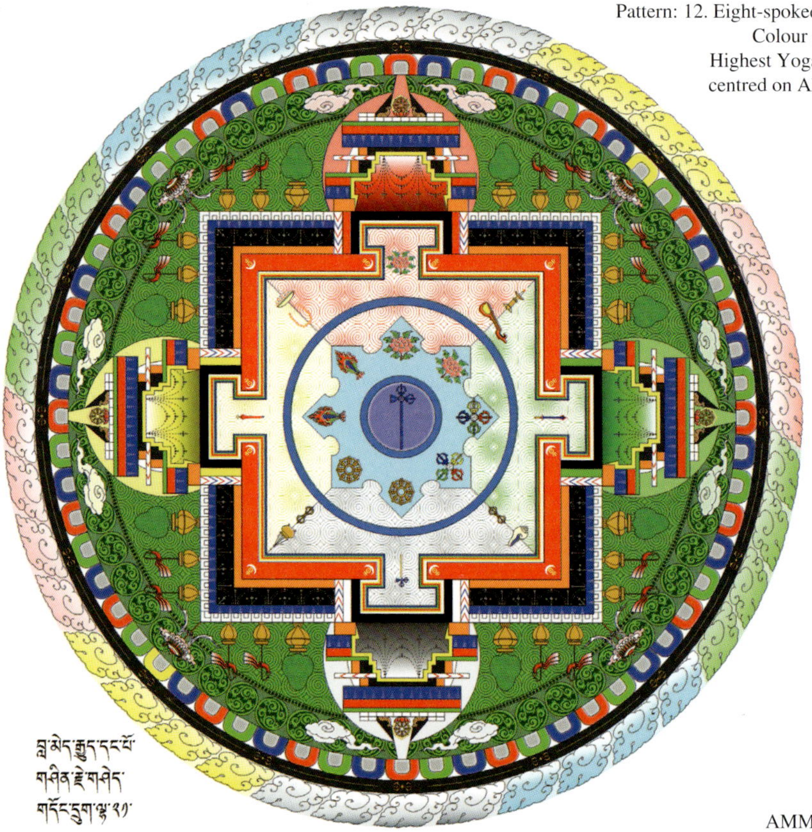

བླ་མེད་རྒྱུད་དང་པོ་
གཤིན་རྗེ་གཤེད་
གདོང་དྲུག་ལྷ་༢༡་

AMM: No. 23

The Highest Yoga tantras in the Hahn Foundation handscroll of the *Mitra brgya rtsa* start with this maṇḍala. It is centred on six-headed Yamāntaka (here represented by a vajra-hammer), a wrathful emanation of Mañjuśrī. It takes the form of an eight-spoked wheel, in the centre of which is the main deity, six-headed, six-armed and six-legged Yamāntaka, red in complexion and accompanied by his consort Vajravetālī. Mohayamāri (east), Matsaryayamāri (south), Rāgayamāri (west) and Īrṣyāyamāri (north) are arranged on the spokes in the four cardinal directions, and on the spokes in the four intermediate directions are the four wrathful goddesses Pṛthivīvajrā (southeast), Abvajrā (southwest), Tejovajrā (northwest) and Vāyuvajrā (northeast). The four inner offering goddesses Lāsyā, Mālā, Gītā and Nṛtyā and the four outer offering goddesses Dhūpā, Puṣpā, Dīpā and Gandhā occupy the four corners of the inner square. In the four gates are the four gatekeepers Mudgarayamāri (east), Daṇḍayamāri (south), Padmayamāri (west) and Khaḍgayamāri (north). It is worth noting that the Hahn Foundation handscroll depicts all the deities by means of their symbols. The colour scheme of the courtyard is that of the Highest Yoga tantras centred on Akṣobhya (Type E). The arrangement of the deities is nearly identical to that of the twenty-one-deity Ṣaṇmukha-Mañjuśrī-Yamāri maṇḍala (No. 53) among the Ṅor maṇḍalas.

42. Thirteen-deity Raktayamāri-maṇḍala

Pattern: 8. Crossed vajra;
Colour scheme:
Highest Yoga tantras
centred on Akṣobhya

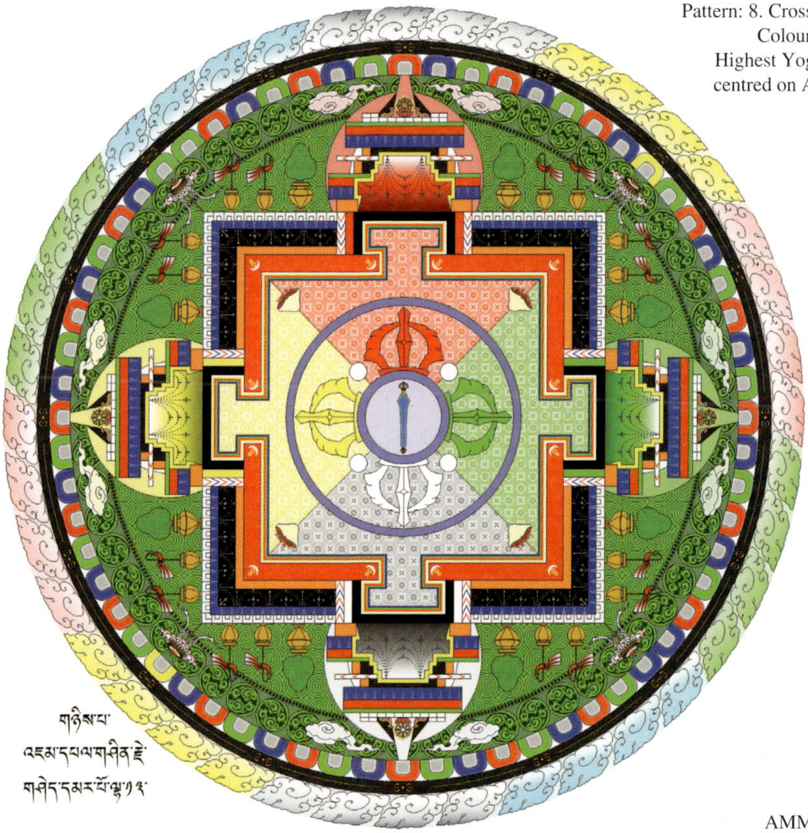

གཉིས་པ་
འཇམ་དཔལ་གཤིན་རྗེ་
གཤེད་དམར་པོ་ལྷ་༡༣་

AMM: No. 24

Raktayamāri means "red enemy of Yama (god of death)" and is thought to be a form of Yamāntaka, the "destroyer of Yama." In Tibet, three styles of Yamāntaka (*gŚin rje dmar nag 'jigs gsum*), namely, Raktayamāri, Kṛṣṇayamāri and Vajrabhairava, are worshipped as the main deity in rites of subjugation (*abhicāraka*) to defeat the enemies of Buddhism. This maṇḍala takes the form of a wheel with four spokes in the shape of a crossed vajra. On the hub of the wheel one-headed and two-armed Raktayamāri (here represented by a blue club) accompanied by his consort Vajravetālī is depicted as the main deity. Mohayamāri (east) together with his consort Carcikā, Matsaryayamāri (south) together with his consort Vārāhī, Rāgayamāri (west) together with his consort Sarasvatī, and Īrṣyāyamāri (north) together with his consort Gaurī are arranged on the spokes in the four cardinal directions. In the four gates are four gatekeepers, starting with Yamarāja. The version in the Hahn Foundation handscroll does not depict any seats for deities on the spokes in the four cardinal directions or in the four gates, and instead it depicts seats between the spokes of the crossed vajra, but this would seem to be a drawing error. The colour scheme of the courtyard is that of the Highest Yoga tantras centred on Akṣobhya (Type E).

43. Nine-deity Vajrabhairava-maṇḍala

Pattern: Nine-panel grid;
Colour scheme:
Highest Yoga tantras
centred on Akṣobhya

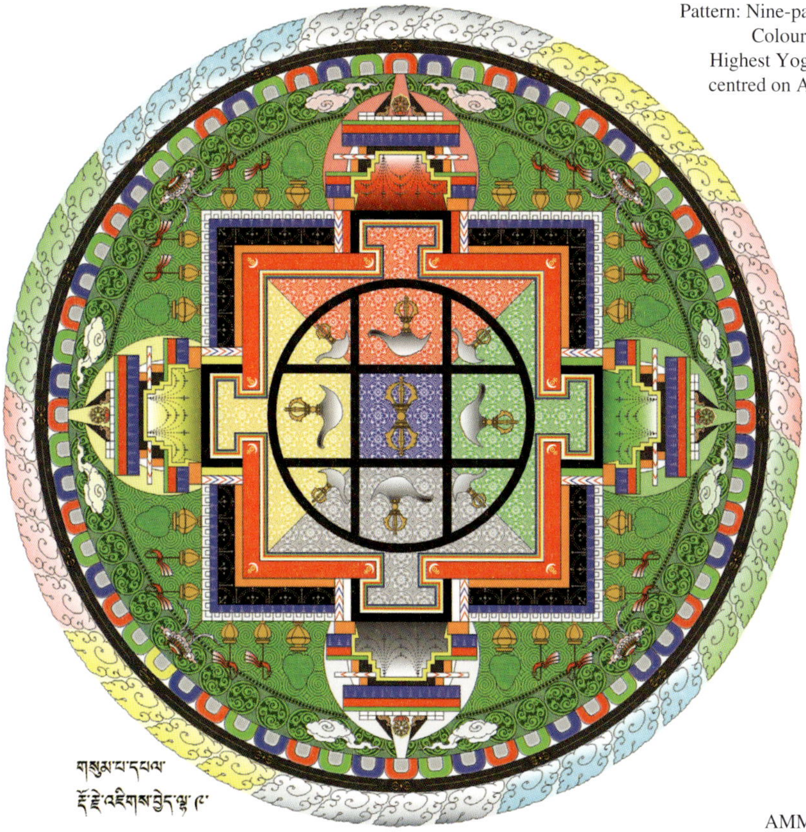

གསུམ་པ་དཔལ་
རྡོ་རྗེ་འཇིགས་བྱེད་ལྷ་༩་

AMM: No. 25

Vajrabhairava is thought to be the most terrifying wrathful deity among the three styles of Yamāntaka (*gŚin rje dmar nag 'jigs gsum*). This maṇḍala takes the form of a nine-panel grid, in the centre of which Vajrabhairava, nine-headed, thirty-two-armed and sixteen-legged, is depicted as the main deity, and he is surrounded by Yamāṅkuśī (east), Yamapāśī (south), Yamasphoṭā (west), Yamāveśā (north), Yamakālarātri (southeast), Yamadūtī (southwest), Daṃṣṭrī (northwest) and Yamadaṇḍī (northeast). The Hahn Foundation handscroll depicts the main deity as a vajra and the eight female attendants as *kartṛ*s (curved knives). In present-day Tibet, especially in the dGe lugs pa order, the thirteen-deity Vajrabhairava maṇḍala, which is consistent with the maṇḍala theory of the *Guhyasamāja-tantra*, is very popular, but the present maṇḍala is rather different. But the seventeen-deity Vajrabhairava-maṇḍala transmitted by sKyo lo tsā ba 'Od zer 'byuṅ gnas (No. 56) among the Ṅor maṇḍalas is quite similar, with the names of the eight attendants almost identical, although it depicts the eight attendants outside the nine-panel grid, and so these two maṇḍalas differ in their arrangement of the deities. Like other maṇḍalas centred on Yamāntaka, the colour scheme of the courtyard is that of the Highest Yoga tantras centred on Akṣobhya (Type E).

44. Eighteen-deity Bhairava-maṇḍala

Pattern: 9. Eight-spoked wheel;
Colour scheme:
Highest Yoga tantras
centred on Akṣobhya

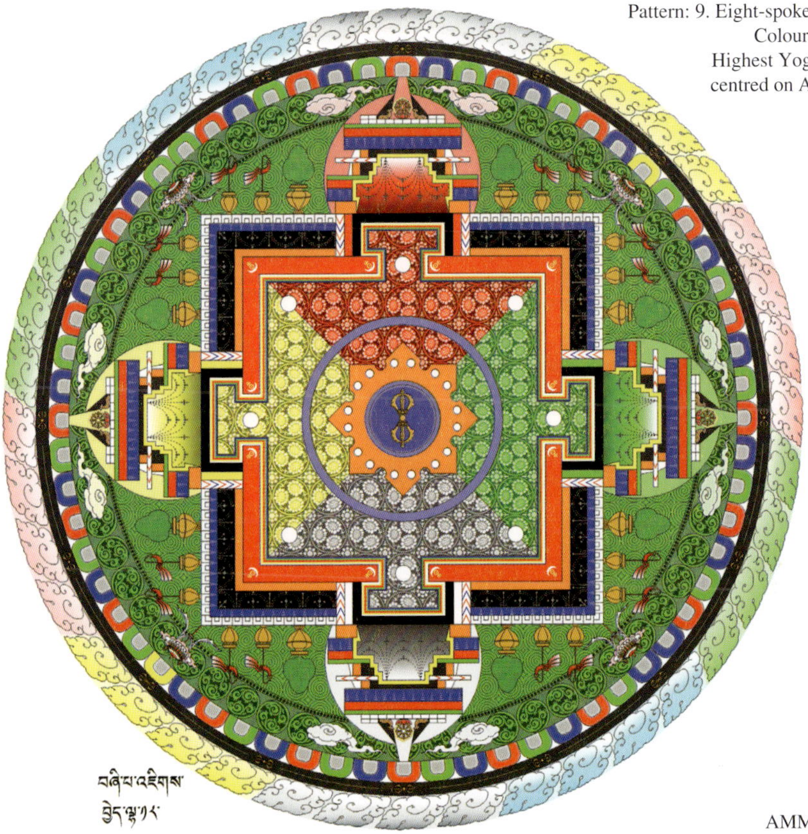

བཞི་པ་འཇིགས་
བྱེད་ལྷ་༡༨་

AMM: No. 26

According to the *Abhisamayamuktāmālā*, this maṇḍala was transmitted by the Indian Tantric practitioner Vairocanarakṣita, who visited Tibet in the twelfth century. It takes the form of an eight-spoked wheel, on the hub of which Vajrabhairava, nine-headed, thirty-four-armed and sixteen-legged (here represented by a vajra), is depicted as the main deity accompanied by his consort Vajravetālī. On the eight spokes are gŚin rje chos kyi rgyal po (east), rTel ba (southeast), A ba glaṅ mgo (south), Ya wa ti (southwest), gŚin rje mig dmar (west), Phya saṅs (northwest), rMig pa (north) and Ral pa tshar dgu (northeast) (Sanskrit names unknown), all of whom are accompanied by consorts. The two circles symbolizing the seats for deities on each of the eight spokes indicate that these eight deities are accompanied by consorts. In the four corners are the four inner offering goddesses Lāsyā, Mālā, Gītā and Nṛtyā, and in the four gates are the four female gatekeepers starting with Aṅkuśī. The seventeen-deity Vajrabhairava-maṇḍala as transmitted by sKyo lo tsā ba 'Od zer 'byuṅ gnas (No. 56) among the Ṅor maṇḍalas is quite similar, with the names of the eight attendants almost identical, but their arrangement differs. Like other maṇḍalas centred on Yamāntaka, the colour scheme of the courtyard is that of the Highest Yoga tantras centred on Akṣobhya (Type E).

45. Nine-deity maṇḍala of two-armed Bhairava

Pattern: 10. Triangle + eight-spoked wheel; Colour scheme: Highest Yoga tantras centred on Akṣobhya

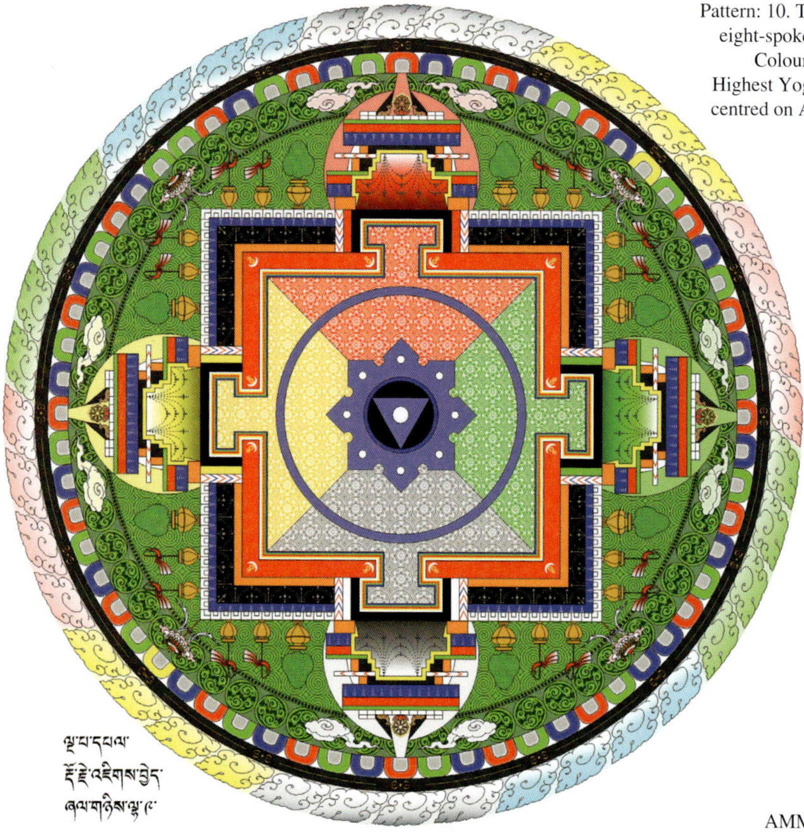

ལྔ་པ་དཔལ་
རྡོ་རྗེ་འཇིགས་བྱེད་
ཞལ་གཉིས་ལྔ་ ༤་

AMM: No. 27

According to the *Abhisamayamuktāmālā*, this maṇḍala is centred on one-headed and two-armed Vajrabhairava, who has the head of a buffalo and holds a *kartṛ* in his right hand and a *kapāla* (skull cup) full of blood in his left hand. It takes the form of a triangle set in an eight-spoked wheel blue-black in colour. In the centre of the triangle, Vajrabhairava is depicted as the main deity. On the eight spokes are the eight attendants gŚin rje ya wa ti (east), Chos rgyal (south), rTel pa (west), A ba glaṅ mgo (north), gŚin rje rmig pa (southeast), Phya saṅs (southwest), Mig dmar (northwest) and Ral pa tshar dgu (northeast). Eight similar attendants also appear in the eighteen-deity Bhairava-maṇḍala (M-44), but their arrangement differs. The inscription of the Hahn Foundation handscroll gives the title of this maṇḍala as "Two-headed Vajrabhairava" (*rDo rje 'jigs byed źal gñis*), but this would seem to be an erroneous abbreviation of "One-headed and two-armed Vajrabhairava" (*rDo rje 'jigs byed źal cig phyag gñis*). Like other maṇḍalas centred on Yamāntaka, the colour scheme of the courtyard is that of the Highest Yoga tantras centred on Akṣobhya (Type E).

46. Fourteen-deity Mahācakravajrapāṇi-maṇḍala

Pattern: 11. Eight petalled lotus + four-spoked wheel; Colour scheme: Highest Yoga tantras centred on Akṣobhya

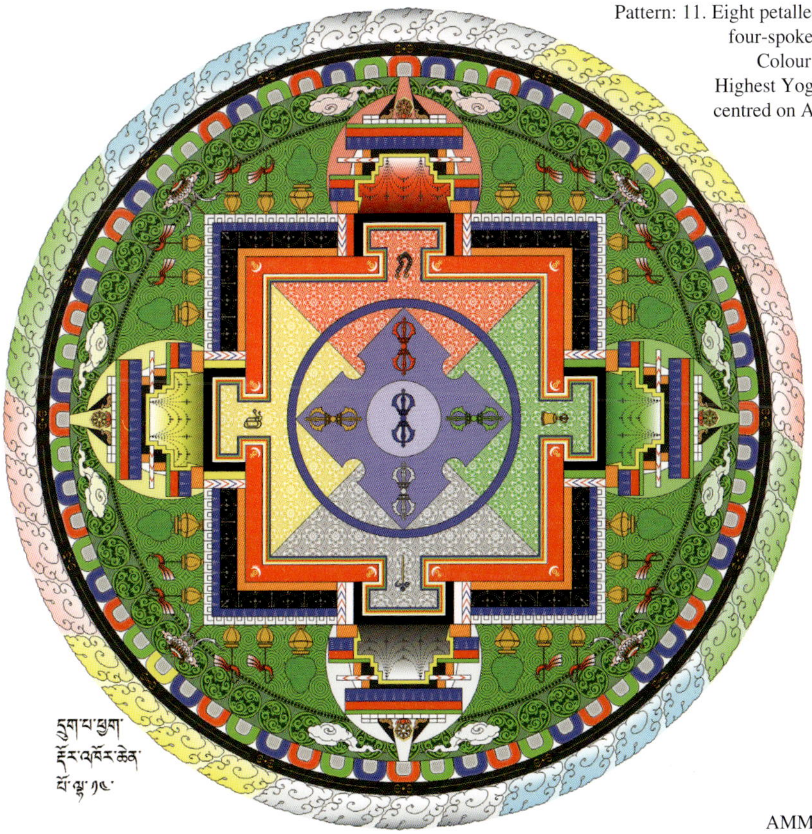

AMM: No. 82

Three-headed and six-armed Mahācakravajrapāṇi, based on the *Nīlāmbaradharavajrapāṇi-tantra*, is a popular tutelary deity in Tibet. His maṇḍala takes the form of a four-spoked wheel, in the centre of which Mahācakravajrapāṇi (here represented by a blue vajra) accompanied by his consort is depicted as the main deity. Surrounding him, on the spokes in the cardinal directions, are the four wrathful deities bDud las rgyal byed (east), rDo rje gzi brjid (south), rṄam pa sgra sgrogs (west) and bDud rtsi 'khyil pa (north) (Sanskrit names unknown), who are all one-headed, four-armed and accompanied by a consort. But in the present example they are represented by vajras in white, yellow, red and green respectively. In the four gates are four pairs of gatekeepers, starting with Aṅkuśa and Aṅkuśī. In some examples, they are depicted as a couple (*yab yum*), while in other examples the male and female deities are positioned on either side of each of the gates. In the Hahn Foundation handscroll, they are represented by symbols, namely, a hook, a noose, a chain and a bell. *Roṅ tha's Iconometry* describes this maṇḍala as an eight-petalled lotus set on the hub of a four-spoked wheel, but many extant examples, including the Hahn Foundation handscroll, omit the eight-petalled lotus. While the total number of deities in this maṇḍala is usually counted as thirteen, the *Padaratnamālā* and the inscription of the Hahn Foundation handscroll include the consort of the main deity, making fourteen deities in all.

47. Twenty-nine-deity maṇḍala of White Saṃvara

Pattern: 13. Triple eight-spoked wheel;
Colour scheme:
Highest Yoga tantras
centred on Akṣobhya

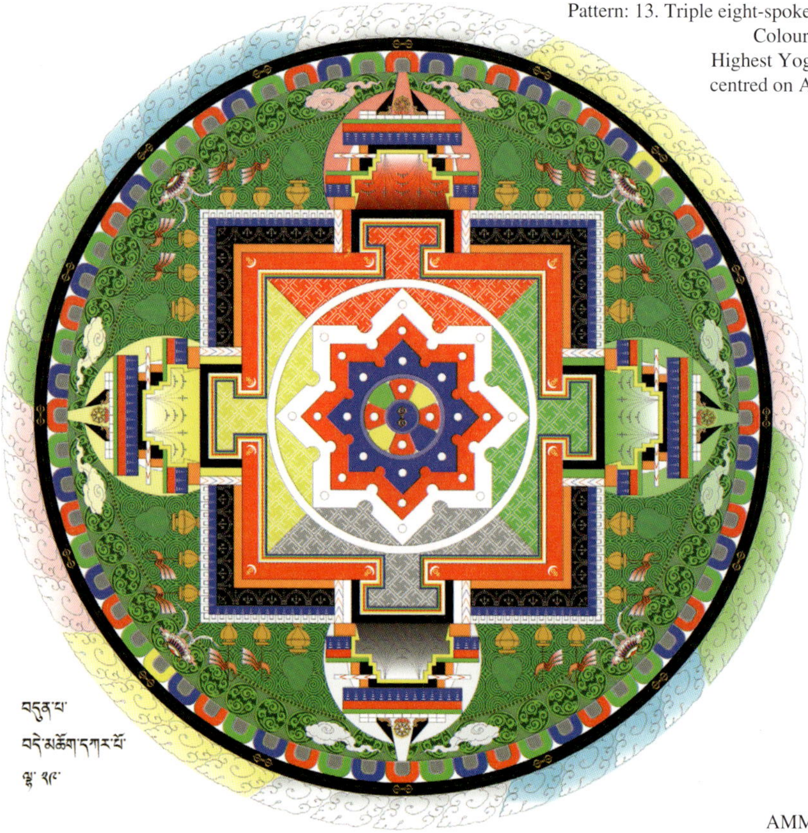

བདུན་པ་
བདེ་མཆོག་དཀར་པོ་
ལྷ་ ༢༩་

AMM: No. 40

The Mother tantras in the Hahn Foundation handscroll of the *Mitra brgya rtsa* start with this maṇḍala. Typical maṇḍalas of the Mother tantras have already been included in the handscroll of the *Vajrāvalī* set, and the handscroll of the *Mitra brgya rtsa* set includes only rare types not included in the *Vajrāvalī* set. Therefore, comments on these maṇḍalas will focus mainly on differences from typical maṇḍalas included in the *Vajrāvalī* set. Like other maṇḍalas belonging to the Saṃvara cycle, this maṇḍala takes the form of a triple eight-spoked wheel around an eight-petalled lotus in the centre. On the pericarp of the lotus, the main deity White Saṃvara is depicted. On the lotus petals in the cardinal directions are the four goddesses Ḍākinī (east), Lāmā (north), Khaṇḍarohā (west) and Rūpiṇī (south). Heroines (female deities) do not appear in this maṇḍala, and only heroes (male deities) are depicted on the wheels of the three mysteries. In addition, the four female animal-headed gatekeepers, starting with Kākāsyā, and the four goddesses starting with Yamaḍāḍhī in the outermost square have been omitted. Thus, the total number of deities is twenty-nine. In this way, this maṇḍala is centred on male deities and is called the "father cycle" (*yab 'khor*). *Roṅ tha's Iconometry* describes this maṇḍala as being identical with other maṇḍalas belonging to the Saṃvara cycle, but the Hahn Foundation handscroll depicts the triple eight-spoked wheel not in the shape of a *dharma-cakra* (wheel of the Law) but in the shape of a *cakra* (wheel) as a weapon.

48. Thirteen-deity Cakrasaṃvara-maṇḍala

Pattern: 16. Eight-petalled lotus;
Colour scheme:
Highest Yoga tantras
centred on Akṣobhya

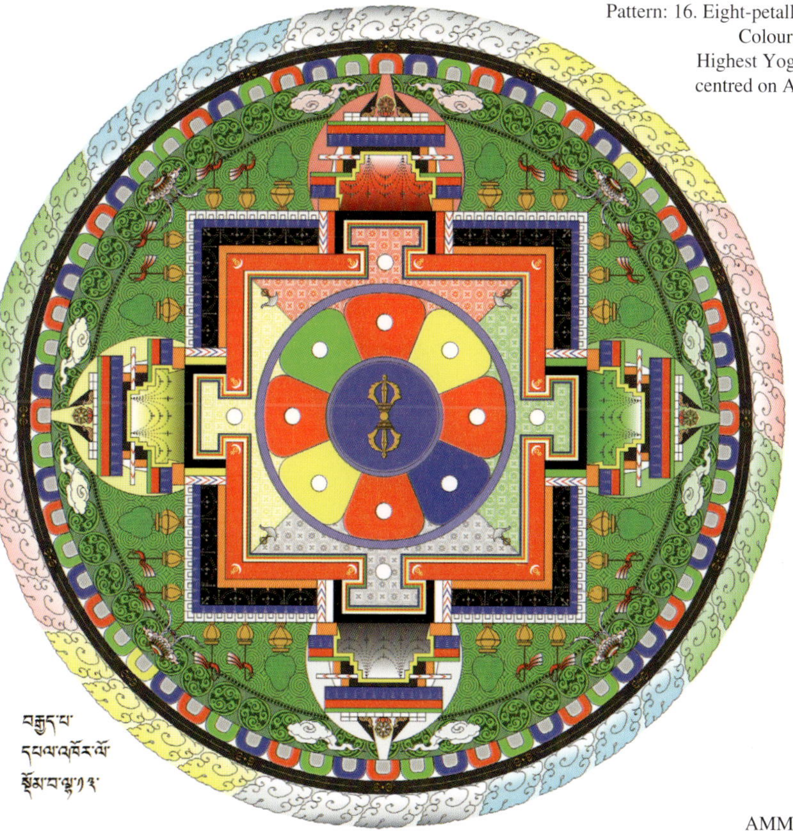

བརྒྱད་པ་
དཔལ་འཁོར་ལོ་
སྡོམ་པ་ལྷ་༡༣་

AMM: No. 42

This maṇḍala takes the form of an eight-petalled lotus, on the pericarp of which four-headed and twelve-armed Saṃvara accompanied by his consort Vajravārāhī is depicted as the main deity. On the lotus petals in the cardinal directions are the four goddesses Ḍākinī (east), Lāmā (north), Khaṇḍarohā (west) and Rūpiṇī (south). In the four gates are the four animal-headed female gatekeepers Kākāsyā (east), Ulūkāsyā (north), Śvānāsyā (west) and Śūkarāsyā (south), while the four goddesses Yamaḍāḍhī (southeast), Yamadūtī (southwest), Yamadaṃṣṭrī (northwest) and Yamamathanī (northeast) (here represented by *kartṛ*s) are arranged in the four corners of the courtyard. This maṇḍala is described in Chapter 13 of the *Saṃvarodaya-tantra,* an explanatory tantra of the Saṃvara cycle, and in composition it corresponds to the sixty-two-deity maṇḍala of Cakrasaṃvara (V-19) minus the circles of the three mysteries of body, speech, and mind. As in other maṇḍalas belonging to the Saṃvara cycle, the colour scheme of the courtyard is that of the Highest Yoga tantras centred on Akṣobhya (Type E). In Tibet, there are not many examples of the thirteen-deity version of the Saṃvara-maṇḍala, whereas in Nepal it is more prevalent.

49. Five-deity Sahajasaṃvara-maṇḍala

Pattern: 16. Eight-petalled lotus;
Colour scheme:
Highest Yoga tantras
centred on Akṣobhya

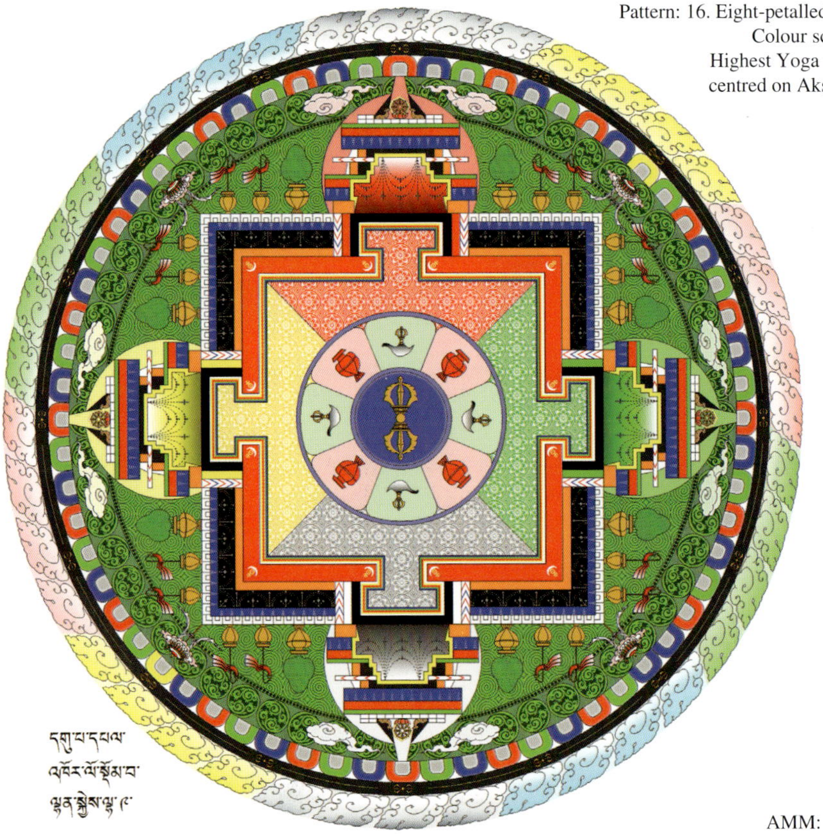

དགུ་པ་དཔལ་
འཁོར་ལོ་སྡོམ་པ་
ལྷན་སྐྱེས་ལྷ་༥་

AMM: No. 43

Sahaja (innate) is a term referring to the ultimate truth of the Mother tantras, while in the iconography of Esoteric Buddhism it signifies the form with which a human being is born, that is, one-headed and two-armed. In Tibetan Buddhism, an image in this style is said to be for those who are unable to visualize a more complex multi-headed and multi-armed image. This maṇḍala takes the form of an eight-petalled lotus, on the pericarp of which one-headed and two-armed Saṃvara accompanied by his consort is depicted as the main deity. On the lotus petals in the cardinal directions the four *ḍākinīs* Vajraḍākinī (east), Karmaḍākinī (north), Padmaḍākinī (west) and Ratnaḍākinī (south) are arranged counterclockwise. As in other maṇḍalas belonging to the Saṃvara cycle, the colour scheme of the courtyard is that of the Highest Yoga tantras centred on Akṣobhya (Type E). This maṇḍala is the simplest among the maṇḍalas belonging to the Saṃvara cycle. However, examples in Tibet are rare, although the main deity Sahajasaṃvara appears frequently in thangkas.

50. Nine-deity Saṃvara-maṇḍala (as transmitted by Tilopa)

Pattern: 16. Eight-petalled lotus;
Colour scheme:
Highest Yoga tantras
centred on Akṣobhya

བཙུ་པ་གྲུབ་ཆེན་ཏེ་ལོ་
པའི་ལུགས་ཀྱི་འཆི་བ་སླུབས་པ་
དཔལ་འཁོར་ལྷ་༩་

AMM: No. 44

Tilopa was an Indian Tantric practitioner who was active from the second half of the tenth century to the first half of the eleventh century. He is one of the patriarchs of the bKa' brgyud pa order of Tibetan Buddhism. This maṇḍala was composed by Tilopa and is thought to be effective for averting unexpected death and extending one's life span. It takes the form of an eight-petalled lotus, on the pericarp of which four-headed and sixteen armed Saṃvara (here represented by a crossed vajra) is depicted as the main deity. The four animal-headed female deities Kākāsyā (east), Ulūkāsyā (north), Śvānāsyā (west) and Śūkarāsyā (south) (here represented by *kartṛ*s) are arranged on the four lotus petals in the cardinal directions surrounding the main deity, while the four goddesses Yamaḍāḍhī (southeast), Yamadūtī (southwest), Yamadaṃṣṭrī (northwest) and Yamamathanī (northeast) (here represented by *kapāla*s) are arranged on the four lotus petals in the intermediate directions. As in other maṇḍalas belonging to the Saṃvara cycle, the colour scheme of the courtyard is that of the Highest Yoga tantras centred on Akṣobhya (Type E). In composition it corresponds to the main deity and the circle of the pledge (*samaya-cakra*) of the sixty-two-deity maṇḍala of Cakrasaṃvara (V-19). Examples of this maṇḍala are rare in Tibet.

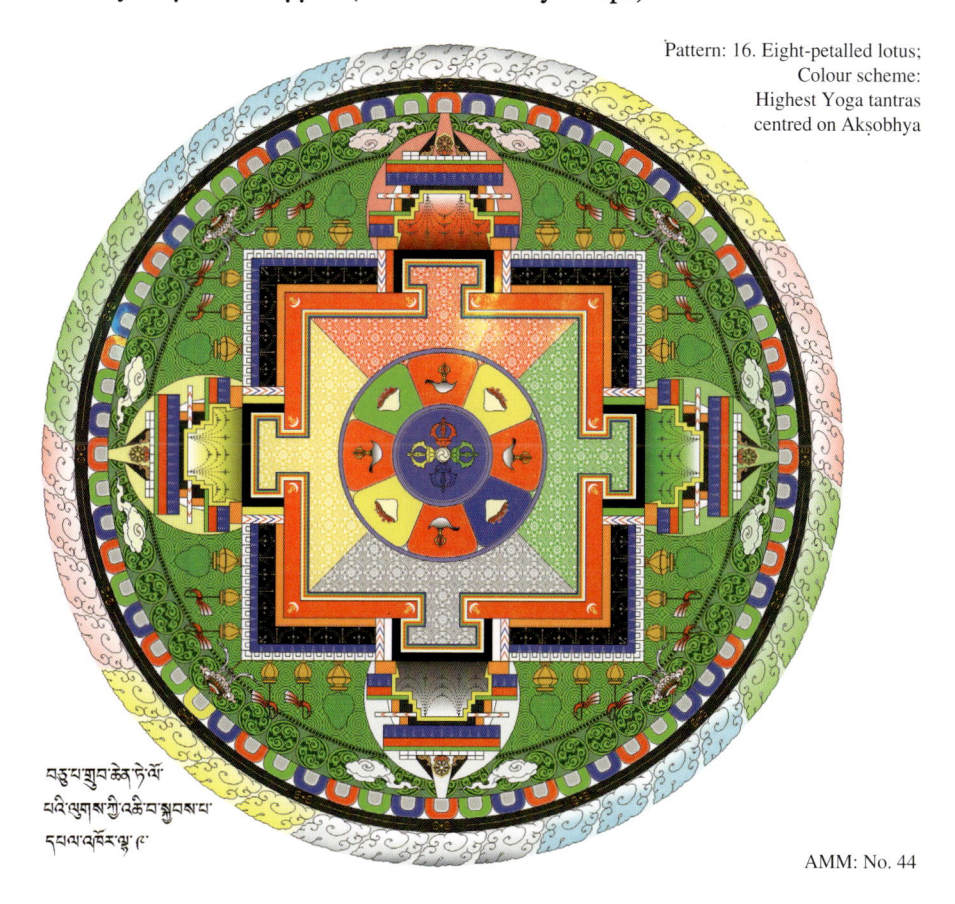

51. Eight-deity Saṃvara-maṇḍala (as transmitted by Advayavajra)

Pattern: 17. Six-spoked wheel;
Colour scheme:
Highest Yoga tantras
centred on Akṣobhya

བཅུ་གཅིག་པ་
གཉིས་མེད་རྡོ་རྗེའི་ལུགས་
ཀྱི་བདེ་མཆོག་ལྷ་བརྒྱད་

AMM: No. 45

The eight-deity Saṃvara-maṇḍala is said to have been composed by Advayavajra, who was an Indian Tantric practitioner active from the end of the tenth century to the middle of the eleventh century and is said to be the same person as Maitrīpa, one of the patriarchs of the bKa' brgyud pa order of Tibetan Buddhism. This maṇḍala takes the form of an unusual six-spoked wheel, on the hub of which three-headed and six-armed Heruka accompanied by his consort (here represented by two small circles) is depicted as the main deity. On the six spokes are Khrag 'thuṅ ma, 'Jigs byed ma, Drag gtum ma, sNaṅ byed ma, rDo rje drag mo and rDo rje mkha' 'gro (Sanskrit names unknown). As in other maṇḍalas belonging to the Saṃvara cycle, the colour scheme of the courtyard is that of the Highest Yoga tantras centred on Akṣobhya (Type E). It is not included in other maṇḍala sets such as the Ṅor maṇḍalas, nor has any coloured thangka depicting this maṇḍala been identified.

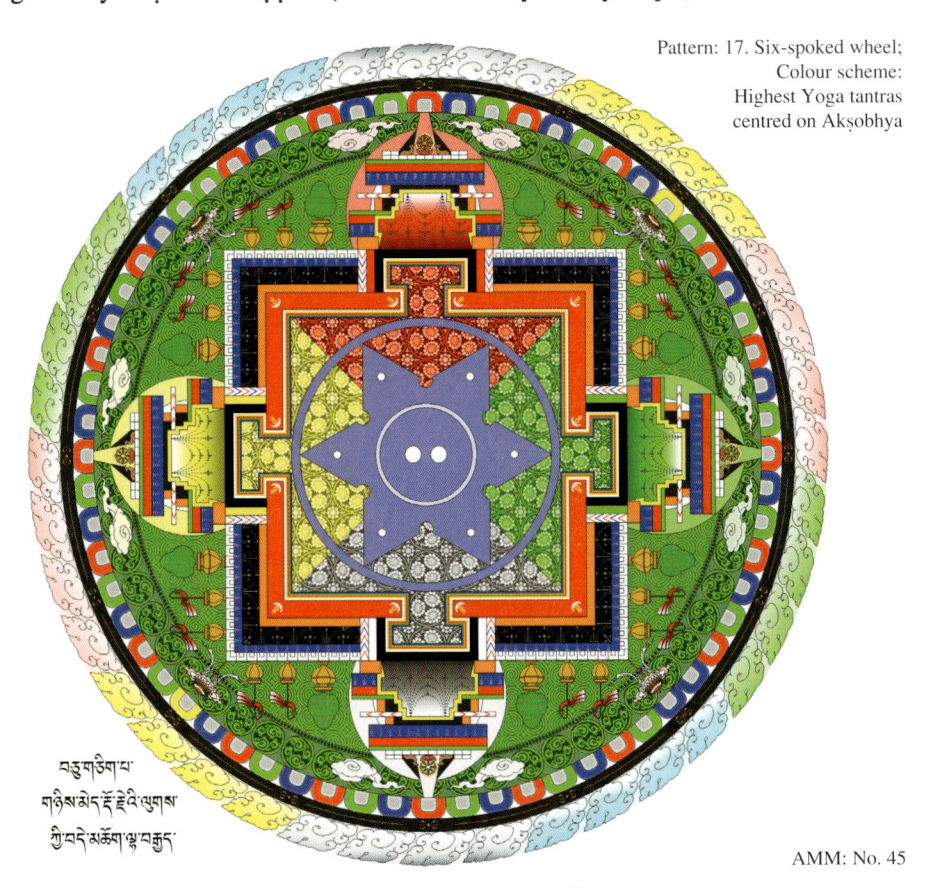

52. Thirteen-deity maṇḍala of three-headed and six-armed Vajravārāhī

Pattern: 16. Eight-petalled lotus;
Colour scheme:
Highest Yoga tantras
centred on Akṣobhya

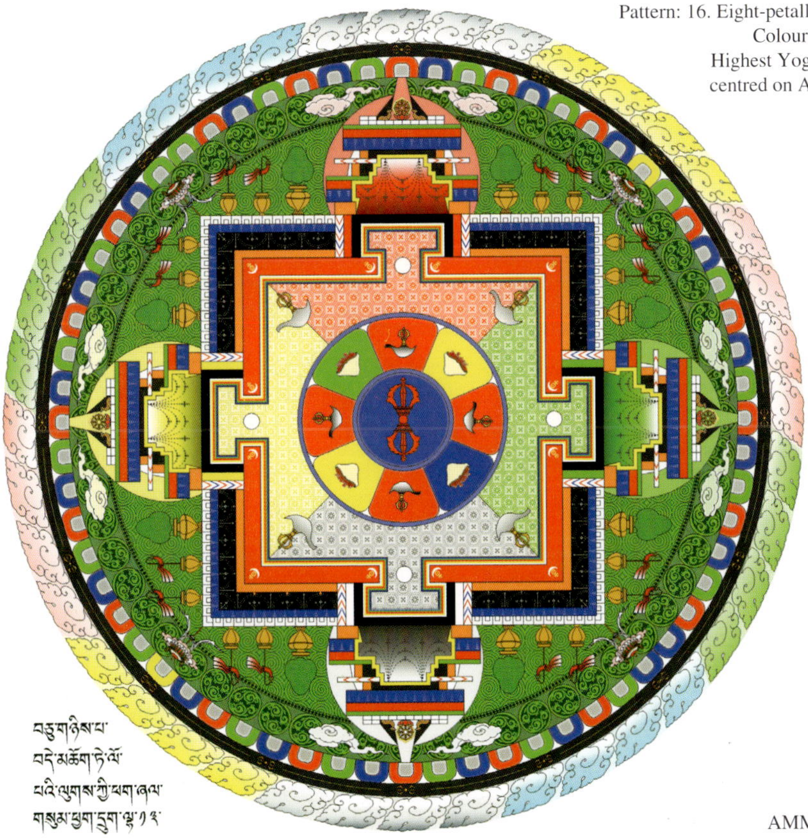

བཅུ་གཉིས་པ་
བདེ་མཆོག་ཏེ་ལོ་
པའི་ལུགས་ཀྱི་ཕག་ཞལ་
གསུམ་ཕྱག་དྲུག་ལྷ་༡༣་

AMM: No. 91

This maṇḍala takes the form of an eight-petalled lotus, on the pericarp of which three-headed and six-armed Vajravārāhī (here represented by a red vajra) is depicted as the main deity. On the lotus petals in the cardinal directions are the four goddesses Ḍākinī (east), Lāmā (north), Khaṇḍarohā (west) and Rūpiṇī (south) (here represented by *kartṛ*s), while *kapāla*s are depicted on the four lotus petals in the intermediate directions. In the four gates are the four animal-headed female gatekeepers Kākāsyā (east), Ulūkāsyā (north), Śvānāsyā (west) and Śūkarāsyā (south), while the four goddesses Yamaḍāḍhī (southeast), Yamadūtī (southwest), Yamadaṃṣṭrī (northwest) and Yamamathanī (northeast) (here represented by *kartṛ*s) are arranged in the four corners of the courtyard. This maṇḍala is thought to be a variant form of the thirteen-deity Cakrasaṃvara-maṇḍala (M-48), in which Saṃvara has been replaced as the main deity by his consort Vajravārāhī. As in other maṇḍalas belonging to the Saṃvara cycle, the colour scheme of the courtyard is that of the Highest Yoga tantras centred on Akṣobhya (Type E).

53. Thirteen-deity maṇḍala of two-headed Vajravārāhī

Pattern: 16. Eight-petalled lotus;
Colour scheme:
Highest Yoga tantras
centred on Akṣobhya

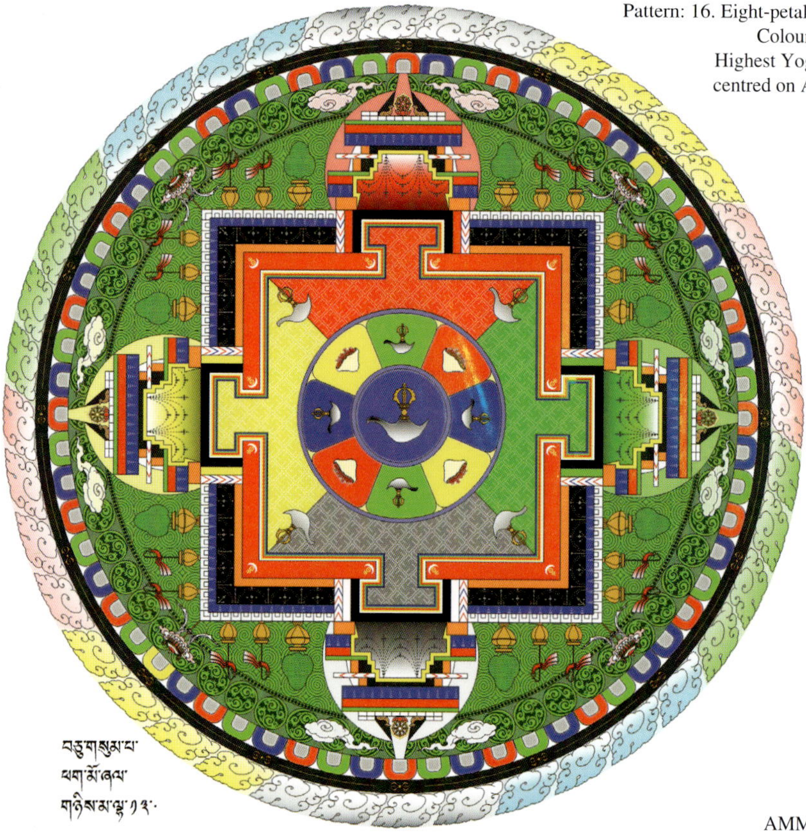

བཅུ་གསུམ་པ་
ཕག་མོ་ཞལ་
གཉིས་མ་ལྔ་༡༣་

AMM: No. 93

Two-headed Vārāhī (Phag mo źal gñis ma) refers to a form of Vajravārāhī who has a face or a protrusion like the face of a wild hog on the right side of her main humanlike face. This maṇḍala takes the form of an eight-petalled lotus, on the pericarp of which two-headed Vajravārāhī (here represented by a *kartṛ*) is depicted as the main deity. On the lotus petals in the cardinal directions are the four goddesses Ḍākinī (east), Lāmā (north), Khaṇḍarohā (west) and Rūpiṇī (south) (here represented by *kartṛ*s), while *kapāla*s are depicted on the four lotus petals in the intermediate directions. In the four gates are the four animal-headed female gatekeepers Kākāsyā (east), Ulūkāsyā (north), Śvānāsyā (west) and Śūkarāsyā (south) (not depicted in the Hahn Foundation handscroll), while the four goddesses Yamaḍāḍhī (southeast), Yamadūtī (southwest), Yamadaṃṣṭrī (northwest) and Yamamathanī (northeast) (here represented by *kartṛ*s) are arranged in the four corners of the courtyard. As in other maṇḍalas belonging to the Saṃvara cycle, the colour scheme of the courtyard is that of the Highest Yoga tantras centred on Akṣobhya (Type E).

54. Thirteen-deity Sarvārthasiddhi-Vārāhī-maṇḍala

Pattern: 16. Eight-petalled lotus;
Colour scheme:
Highest Yoga tantras
centred on Akṣobhya

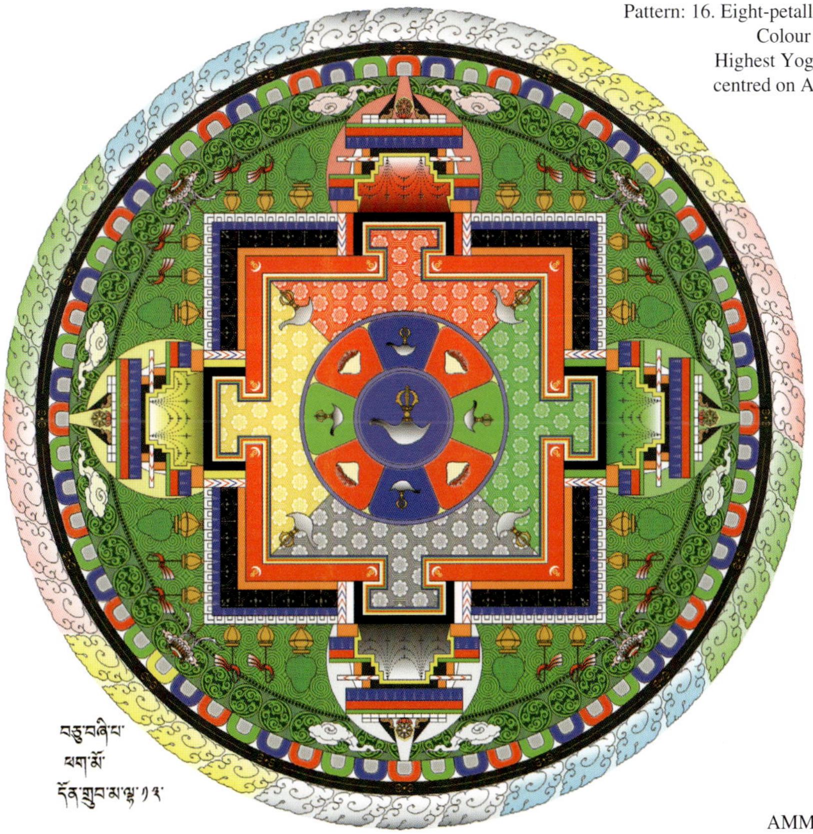

བཅུ་བཞི་པ་
ཕག་མོ་
དོན་གྲུབ་མ་ལྷ་༡༣་

AMM: No. 94

This maṇḍala takes the form of an eight-petalled lotus, on the pericarp of which one-headed and four-armed Vajravārāhī (here represented by a *kartṛ*) is depicted as the main deity. On the lotus petals in the cardinal directions are the four goddesses Ḍākinī (east), Lāmā (north), Khaṇḍarohā (west) and Rūpiṇī (south) (here represented by *kartṛ*s), while *kapāla*s are depicted on the four lotus petals in the intermediate directions. In the four gates are the four animal-headed female gatekeepers Kākāsyā (east), Ulūkāsyā (north), Śvānāsyā (west) and Śūkarāsyā (south) (not depicted in the Hahn Foundation handscroll), while the four goddesses Yamaḍāḍhī (southeast), Yamadūtī (southwest), Yamadaṃṣṭrī (northwest) and Yamamathanī (northeast) (here represented by *kartṛ*s) are arranged in the four corners of the courtyard. As in other maṇḍalas belonging to the Saṃvara cycle, the colour scheme of the courtyard is that of the Highest Yoga tantras centred on Akṣobhya (Type E). This maṇḍala has almost the same structure as the previous maṇḍala (M-53). A hook and a noose, the attributes held in the two additional hands of the main deity, are thought to symbolize the efficacy of this maṇḍala, which "accomplishes all objectives" (*sarvārthasiddhi*).

55. Thirteen-deity Chinnamastakā-Vārāhī-maṇḍala

Pattern: 16. Eight-petalled lotus;
Colour scheme:
Highest Yoga tantras
centred on Akṣobhya

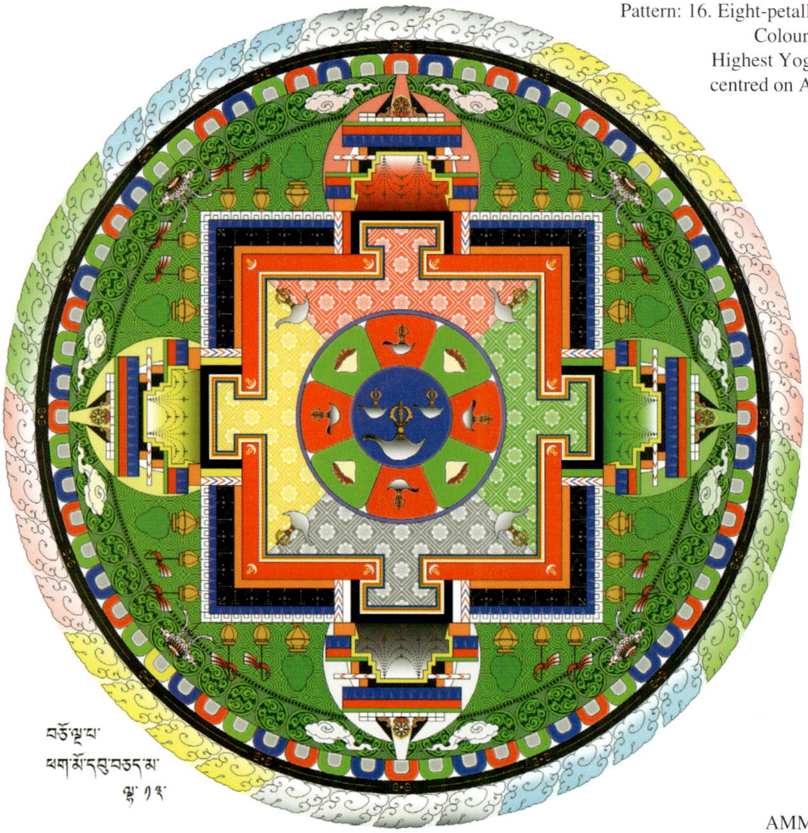

བཅོ་ལྔ་པ་
ཕག་མོ་དབུ་བཅད་མ་
ལྷ་ ༡༣

AMM: No. 95

Chinnamastakā means "the beheaded one" and refers to a headless form of the Hindu goddess Durgā who drinks from a stream of blood flowing from her own decapitated body. Tantric Buddhism, on the other hand, regarded her as a form of Vajravārāhī, the consort of Cakrasaṃvara. Her maṇḍala takes the form of an eight-petalled lotus, on the pericarp of which Chinnamastakā (here represented by a *kartṛ*) is depicted as the main deity. On the lotus petals in the cardinal directions are the four goddesses Ḍākinī (east), Lāmā (north), Khaṇḍarohā (west) and Rūpiṇī (south) (here represented by *kartṛ*s), while *kapāla*s are depicted on the four lotus petals in the intermediate directions. Two small *kartṛ*s placed on both sides of the main deity symbolize two female attendants of Chinnamastakā. In the four gates are the four animal-headed female gatekeepers starting with Kākāsyā (not depicted in the Hahn Foundation handscroll), while the four goddesses starting with Yamaḍāḍhī (here represented by *kartṛ*s) are arranged in the four corners of the courtyard. As in other maṇḍalas belonging to the Saṃvara cycle, the colour scheme of the courtyard is that of the Highest Yoga tantras centred on Akṣobhya (Type E). Because of her extraordinary appearance, Chinnamastakā was not welcomed in Tibet, but in Nepal many examples of her image can be seen even today.

56. Thirteen-deity Vārāhī-maṇḍala (as transmitted by Nāropa)

Pattern: 3. hexagram like the Star of David;
Colour scheme: Highest Yoga tantras centred on Akṣobhya

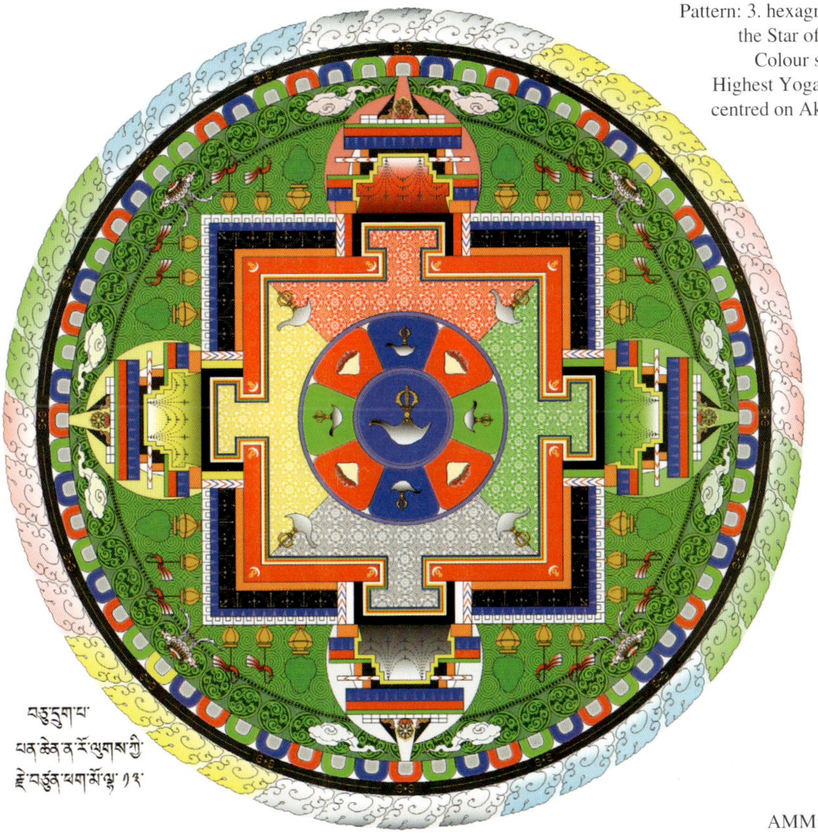

བཅུ་དྲུག་པ་
པཎ་ཆེན་ན་རོ་ལུགས་ཀྱི་
རྡོ་རྗེ་བཙུན་ཕག་མོ་ལྷ་༡༣་

AMM: No. 92

Nāropa was an Indian Tantric practitioner who was active from the end of the tenth century to the middle of the eleventh century, and he is one of the patriarchs of the bKa' brgyud pa order of Tibetan Buddhism. The maṇḍala of Vajravārāhī attributed to Nāropa takes the form of an eight-petalled lotus, on the pericarp of which Vajravārāhī (here represented by a *kartṛ*) is depicted as the main deity. On the lotus petals in the cardinal directions are the four goddesses starting with Ḍākinī (here represented by *kartṛ*s), while *kapāla*s are depicted on the four lotus petals in the intermediate directions. In the four gates are the four animal-headed female gatekeepers starting with Kākāsyā (not depicted in the Hahn Foundation handscroll), while the four goddesses starting with Yamaḍāḍhī (here represented by *kartṛ*s) are arranged in the four corners of the courtyard. Among maṇḍalas belonging to the "mother cycle" (*yum 'khor*) of the Mother tantras, examples of this maṇḍala are common in Tibet. *Roṅ tha's Iconometry* describes this maṇḍala as a hexagram similar to the Star of David, and many extant examples match this description. But it is worth noting that the Hahn Foundation handscroll adopts an eight-petalled lotus in accordance with the *Abhisamayamuktāmālā*. As in other maṇḍalas belonging to the Saṃvara cycle, the colour scheme of the courtyard is that of the Highest Yoga tantras centred on Akṣobhya (Type E).

57. Nine-deity Ḍākinī-maṇḍala (as transmitted by Maitrīpa)

Pattern: 18b. Eight-spoked wheel;
Colour scheme:
Highest Yoga tantras
centred on Akṣobhya

བཅུ་བདུན་པ་
མཻ་ཏྲི་མཁའ་སྤྱོད་
མ་ལྷ་༩་

AMM: No. 97

Maitrīpa was an Indian Tantric practitioner who was active from the end of the tenth century to the first half of the eleventh century, and he is one of the patriarchs of the bKa' brgyud pa order of Tibetan Buddhism. Vajravārāhī as attributed to him was called "Maitrīpa's *ḍākinī*" (*Maitri mkha' spyod*) in Tibet, and her iconographical characteristic is her left foot raised to the level of her shoulder. This maṇḍala takes the form of an eight-spoked wheel, on the hub of which Maitrīpa's *ḍākinī* (here represented by a vajra) is depicted as the main deity. On the spokes in the eight directions are the eight goddesses rDo rje mkha' 'gro, gŚin rje mo, Yid bźin mo, sMoṅs byed mo, dBaṅ bsdud ma, Kun skyod ma, Kun grags ma and gTum mo (Sanskrit names unknown). In Tibet, Maitrīpa's *ḍākinī* is frequently included in compendia of iconography, but her maṇḍala is not included in any other maṇḍala sets, and examples of coloured thangkas are rare.

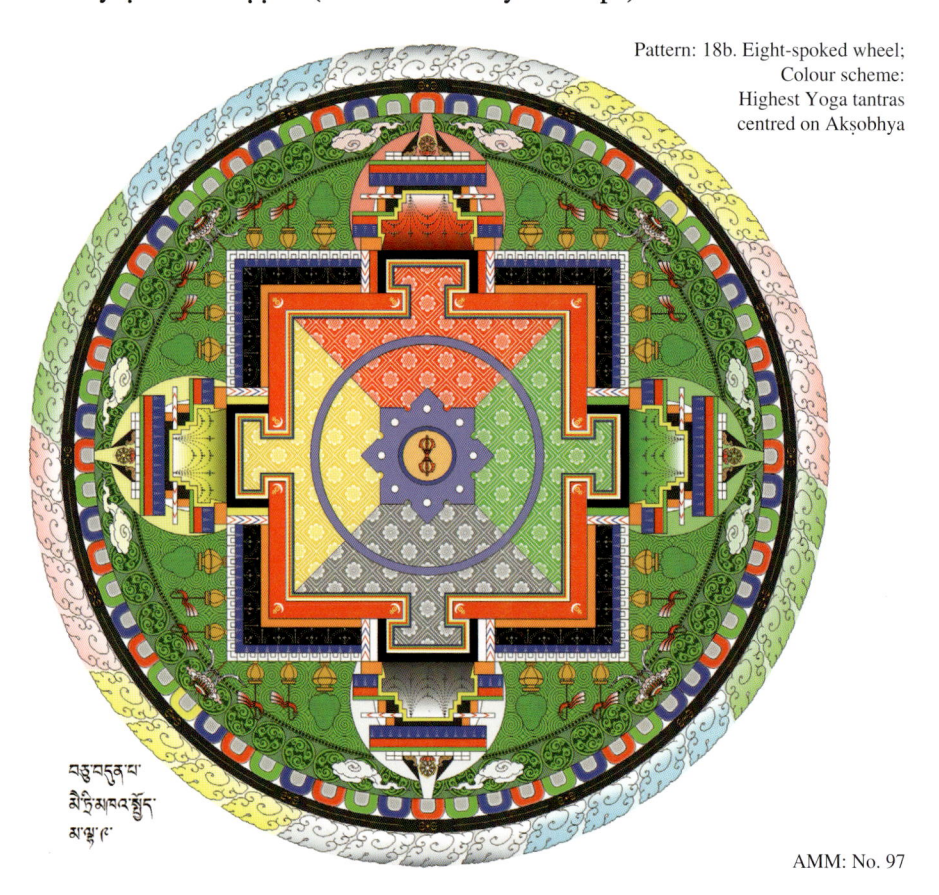

58. Thirty-seven-deity maṇḍala of four-headed Vārāhī

Pattern: 13. Triple eight-spoked wheel;
Colour scheme:
Highest Yoga tantras centred on Akṣobhya

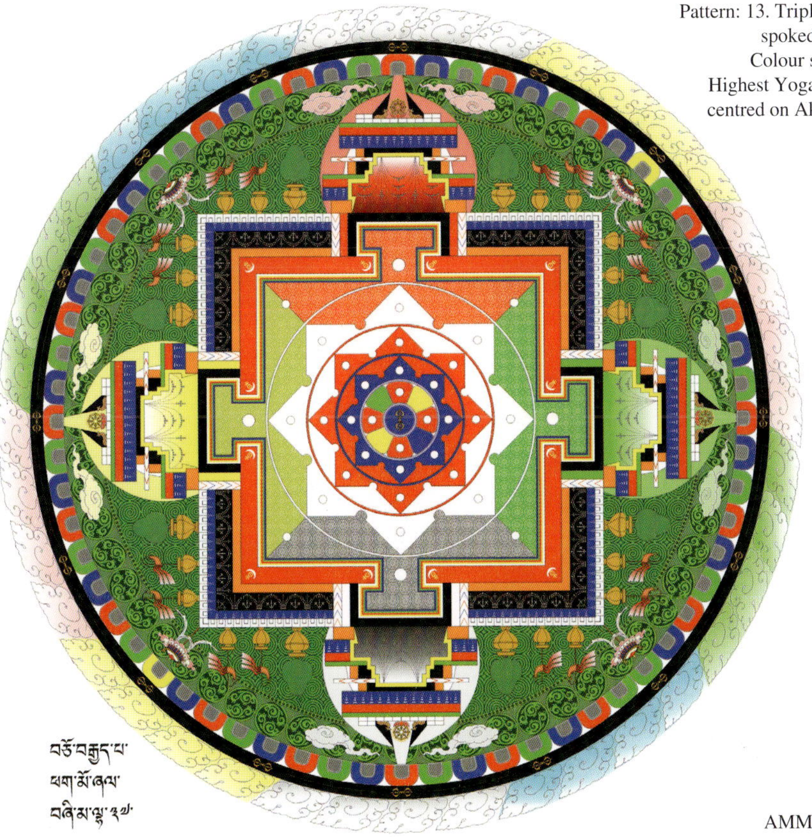

བཅོ་བརྒྱད་པ་
ཕག་མོ་ཞལ་
བཞི་མ་ལྷ་༣༧་

AMM: No. 98

Like the sixty-two-deity Cakrasaṃvara-maṇḍala (V-19), this maṇḍala takes the form of a triple eight-spoked wheel surrounding an eight-petalled lotus, in the centre of which four-headed and twelve-armed Vajravārāhī (here represented by a vajra) is depicted as the main deity. On the lotus petals in the cardinal directions are the four goddesses Ḍākinī (east), Lāmā (north), Khaṇḍarohā (west) and Rūpiṇī (south). On the wheels of the three mysteries only *yoginī*s (female deities) are depicted, and on the wheel of the pledge (*samaya-cakra*) the four animal-headed female gatekeepers Kākāsyā (east), Ulūkāsyā (north), Śvānāsyā (west) and Śūkarāsyā (south) and the four goddesses Yamaḍāḍhī (southeast), Yamadūtī (southwest), Yamadaṃṣṭrī (northwest) and Yamamathanī (northeast) are arranged. Thus, the total number of deities is thirty-seven. As in the twenty-nine-deity maṇḍala of White Saṃvara (M-47), the Hahn Foundation handscroll depicts a triple eight-spoked wheel not in the shape of a *dharma-cakra* but in the shape of a *cakra* as a weapon. As in other maṇḍalas belonging to the Saṃvara cycle, the colour scheme of the courtyard is that of the Highest Yoga tantras centred on Akṣobhya (Type E).

59. Five-deity maṇḍala of Black Vārāhī

Pattern: 18a. Four-spoked wheel;
Colour scheme: Highest
Yoga tantras centred
on Akṣobhya

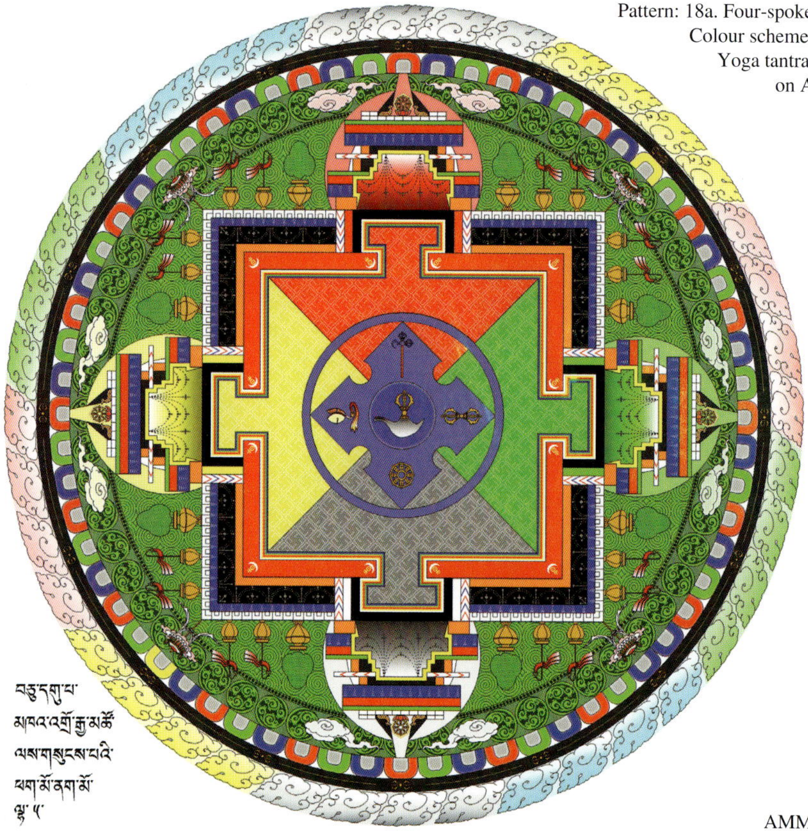

བཅུ་དགུ་པ་
མཁའ་འགྲོ་རྒྱ་མཚོ་
ལས་གསུངས་པའི་
ཕག་མོ་ནག་མོ་
ལྷ་ ༥་

AMM: No. 96

Vajravārāhī, the consort of Saṃvara and the main deity of the "mother cycle" (*yum 'khor*) of Saṃvara, usually has a red complexion, but a variant form black in colour is called Black Vārāhī. Her maṇḍala takes the form of a four-spoked wheel, on the hub of which one-headed and two-armed Black Vārāhī (here represented by a *kartṛ*) is depicted as the main deity. On the lotus petals in the four cardinal directions are Rohī (east; represented by a wheel), Khaṇḍarohī (south; represented by a *ḍamaru* [hand drum]), Bhūcarī (west; represented by a hook) and Khecarī (north; represented by a vajra). As in other maṇḍalas belonging to the Saṃvara cycle, the colour scheme of the courtyard is that of the Highest Yoga tantras centred on Akṣobhya (Type E). The maṇḍala of Black Vārāhī is not included in any other maṇḍala sets, nor has any coloured thangka depicting this maṇḍala been identified. But there is a coloured thangka depicting Black Vārāhī and four female attendants in a private collection in Japan.

60. Five-deity Mahāmāyā-maṇḍala (medium)

Pattern: 16. Eight-petalled lotus;
Colour scheme:
Highest Yoga tantras
centred on Akṣobhya

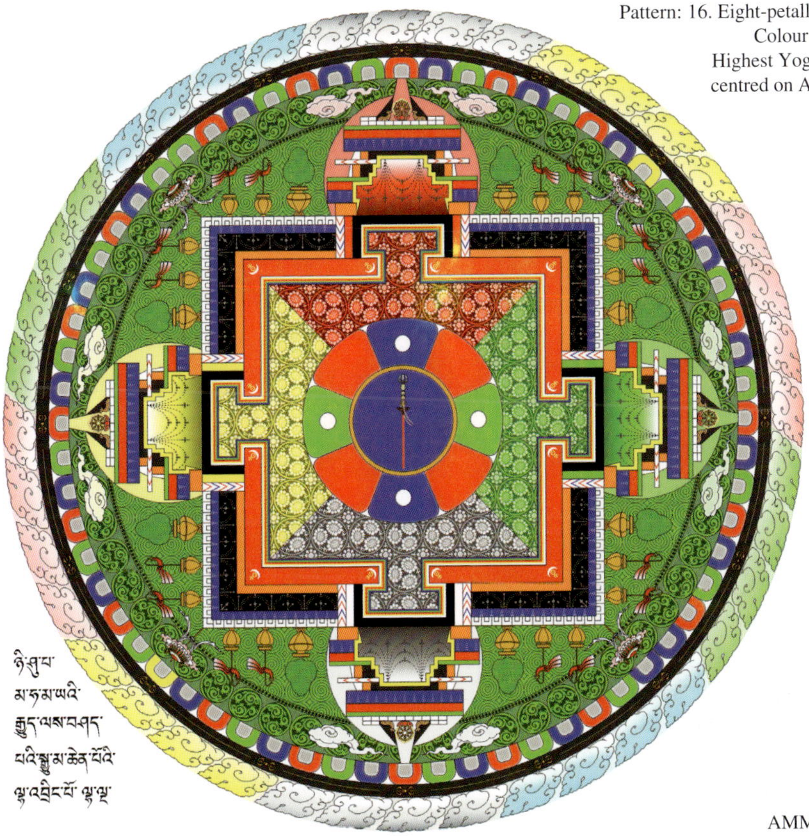

ཉེ་ཤུ་པ་
མ་ཧ་མ་ཡའི་
རྒྱུད་ལས་བཤད་
པའི་སྒྱུ་མ་ཆེན་པོའི་
ལྷ་འབྲིང་པོ་ ལྷ་ལྔ་

AMM: No. 59

The *Mahāmāyā-tantra* is one of the Mother tantras of the Highest Yoga tantras, and Heruka, the main deity of this tantra, is usually called Mahāmāyā. The *Abhisamayamuktāmālā* describes three kinds of Mahāmāyā-maṇḍala, large, medium and small, and this maṇḍala corresponds to the medium version. It takes the form of an eight-petalled lotus, on the pericarp of which is depicted as the main deity one-headed and two-armed Mahāmāyā (here represented by a *khaṭvāṅga*), who holds a *khaṭvāṅga* and a *kapāla* and is accompanied by his consort. On the lotus petals in the cardinal directions are Vajraḍākinī (east), Viśvaḍākinī (north), Padmaḍākinī (west) and Ratnaḍākinī (south). The inscription of the Hahn foundation handscroll gives the number of deities as five, while the *Padaratnamālā* includes the consort of the main deity, making a total of six. Unlike the other two maṇḍalas centred on Mahāmāyā (V-33 and M-61), the colour scheme of the courtyard is that of the Highest Yoga tantras centred on Akṣobhya (Type E).

61. Five-deity Mahāmāyā-maṇḍala (small)

Pattern: 22. Four-petalled lotus;
Colour scheme:
Yoga tantras centred
on Vairocana

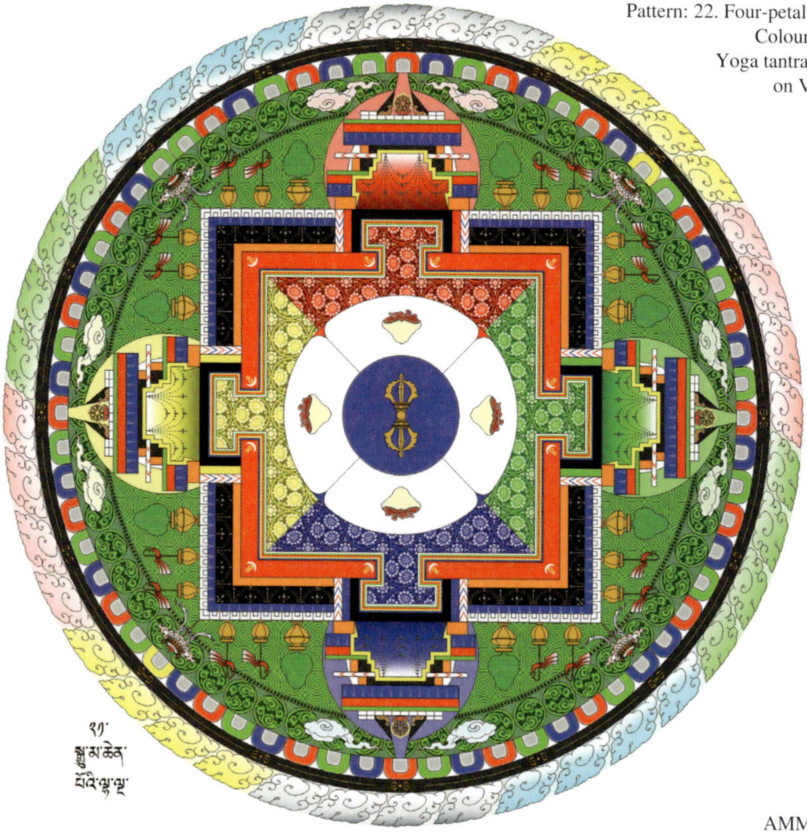

༦༡་
སྒྱུ་མ་ཆེན་
པོའི་ལྷ་ལྔ་

AMM: No. 60

The *Mahāmāyā-tantra* is one of the Mother tantras of the Highest Yoga tantras, and the main deity of this tantra is usually called Mahāmāyā. But because Mahāmāyā is a feminine noun, according to some scholars the masculine form Mahāmāya is correct. The *Abhisamayamuktāmālā* describes three kinds of Mahāmāyā-maṇḍala, large, medium and small, and this maṇḍala corresponds to the small version. It takes the form of a white four-petalled lotus, on the pericarp of which is depicted as the main deity one-headed and two-armed Vajrasattva (here represented by a vajra), who is embracing his consort by crossing both arms and holds a vajra and a bell in his two hands. On the lotus petals in the four cardinal directions are arranged not deities but four *kapāla*s. The *Abhisamayamuktāmālā* and *Roṅ tha's Iconometry* describe this maṇḍala as a single-deity maṇḍala, whereas the inscription of the Hahn Foundation handscroll also counts the four *kapāla*s as deities, making a total of five, but this would seem unwarranted. Like the six-deity Mahāmāyā-maṇḍala (V-33) in the *Vajrāvalī* set, the colour scheme of the courtyard is that of the Yoga tantras centred on Vairocana (Type A).

62. Thirteen-deity Jinasāgara-maṇḍala

Pattern: 16. Eight-petalled lotus;
Colour scheme:
Yoga tantras centred
on Vairocana

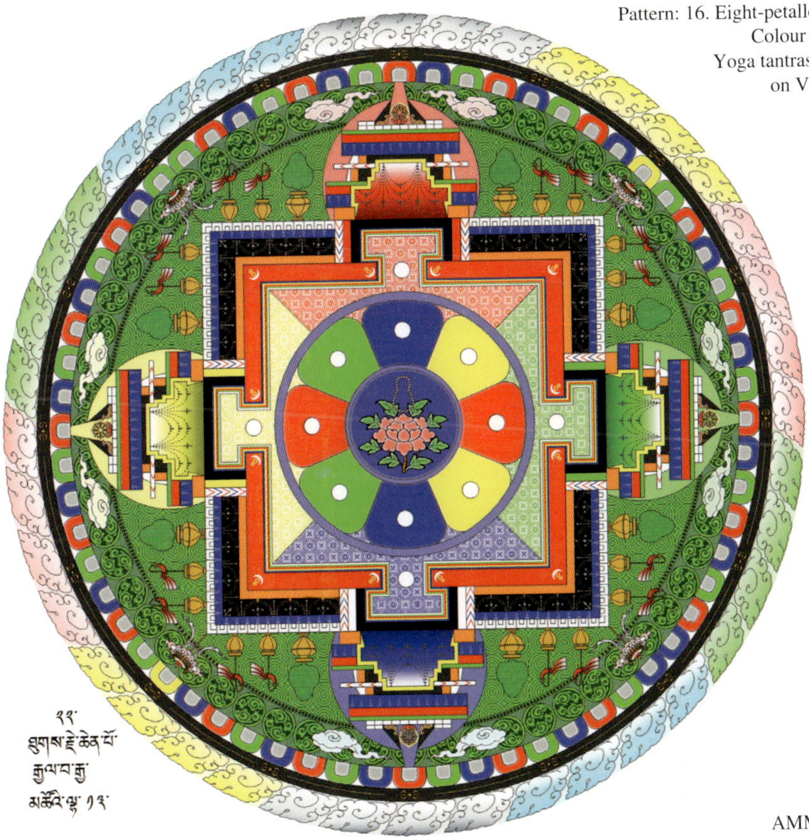

༨༨་
ཐུགས་རྗེ་ཆེན་པོ་
རྒྱལ་བ་རྒྱ་
མཚོའི་ལྷ་ ༡༣་

AMM: No. 88

Jinasāgara, a form of Avalokiteśvara belonging to the Highest Yoga tantras, is widely worshipped in Tibet. According to the *Abhisamayamuktāmālā*, this maṇḍala takes the form of an eight-petalled lotus, on the pericarp of which is depicted as the main deity one-headed and two-armed Jinasāgara (here represented by a rosary and a lotus), who is embracing his consort Jñānaḍākinī with both hands, in which he holds a rosary of pearls (right) and a blue lotus (*utpala*) (left). On the lotus petals in the four cardinal directions are Vajraḍākinī (east), Ratnaḍākinī (south), Padmaḍākinī (west) and Karmaḍākinī (north), while on the lotus petals in the four intermediate directions the messengers (*giṅ*) of the Vajra, Jewel, Lotus and Action families are arranged. Jinasāgara, the main deity of this maṇḍala, is included in several compendia of iconography. However, his iconography is not fixed, and several variations are known to exist, e.g., two-armed, four-armed, accompanied by a consort, and without a consort. The colour scheme of the courtyard is that of the Yoga tantras centred on Vairocana (Type A) even though the main deity belongs to the Lotus family presided over by Amitābha. This colour scheme seems to have been chosen to accord with the arrangement of the four *ḍākinī*s in the four cardinal directions.

63. Eighteen-deity Hayagrīva-Padmanarteśvara-maṇḍala

Pattern: 16. Eight-petalled lotus;
Colour scheme:
Highest Yoga tantras
centred on Amitābha

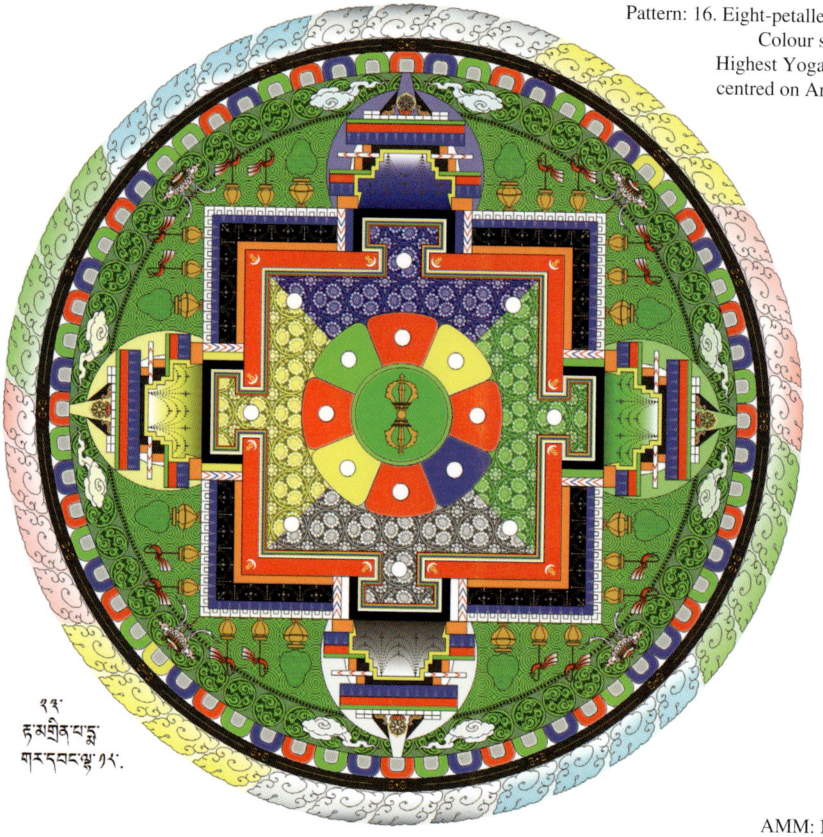

༦༣་
རྟ་མགྲིན་པ་དྨ་
གར་དབང་ལྷ་༡༨་

AMM: No. 77

Padmanarteśvara is the main deity of the Padmanarteśvara clan, one of the six clans of the Mother tantras of the Highest Yoga tantras. The Padmanarteśvara clan corresponds to the Lotus family of the Yoga tantras and the Father tantras of the Highest Yoga tantras, and the *Abhisamayamuktāmālā* considers Padmanarteśvara and Hayagrīva to be the same deity. This maṇḍala takes the form of an eight-petalled lotus, on the pericarp of which Padmanarteśvara, three-headed and eight-armed, is depicted being embraced by his consort Pāṇḍarā. On the eight lotus petals are the eight goddesses Vilokinī (east), Vajrasattvā (southeast), Īśvarī (south), Ratnasattvā (southwest), Bhṛkuṭī (west), Padmasattvā (northwest), Tārā (north) and Viśvā (northeast). These eight goddesses include three attendants of the Padmanarteśvara clan mentioned in the *Sarvabuddhasamāyoga-tantra,* an early Mother tantra which first introduced the six-clan system. In the four corners of the courtyard are the four outer offering goddesses Dhūpā, Puṣpā, Dīpā and Gandhā, and in the four gates are the four female gatekeepers Aṅkuśī, Pāśī, Sphoṭā and Ghaṇṭā. Thus, the total number of deities, including Pāṇḍarā, the consort of the main deity, is eighteen. The colour scheme of the courtyard is that of the Highest Yoga tantras centred on Amitābha (Type F) since the Padmanarteśvara clan corresponds to the Lotus family presided over by Amitābha.

64. Maṇḍala of twenty-one types of Tārā (as transmitted by Sūryagupta)

Pattern: 21. Four-petalled lotus + eight-petalled lotus;
Colour scheme: Highest Yoga tantras centred on Akṣobhya

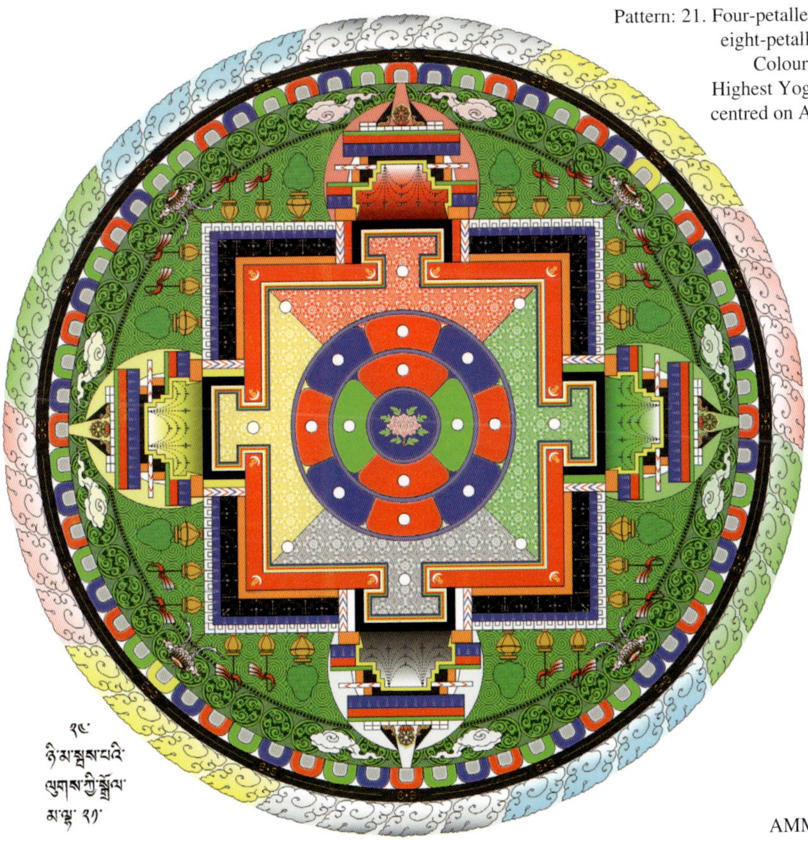

༢༩་
ཉི་མ་སྦས་པའི་
ལུགས་ཀྱི་སྒྲོལ་
མ་ལྷ་ ༢༡་

AMM: No. 99

The twenty-one types of Tārā (*sGrol ma ñer gcig*) are based on the *Ekaviṃśati-stotra* of Tārā. This work consists of twenty-one Sanskrit hymns praising various virtues of Tārā. Later, twenty-one images were created in accordance with the virtues described in each of the hymns. Their iconography adopts one of two styles: the Atīśa style, in which all the images have a single head and two arms, and the Sūryagupta style, in which all the images are multi-headed and multi-armed, all different from each other. This maṇḍala is based on the Sūryagupta tradition. The centre of the maṇḍala takes the form of a combination of a four-petalled lotus and an eight-petalled lotus, and on the pericarp of the four-petalled lotus one-headed and eight-armed Tārā (here represented by a red lotus) is depicted as the main deity. The emanations of Tārā are arranged on the lotus petals of the inner four-petalled and outer eight-petalled lotus, in the four corners of the courtyard, and in the four gates. Thus, the total number of emanations is twenty-one. The names of the twenty-one types of Tārā are not given in the *Abhisamayamuktāmālā*, but the iconography of the main deity which it describes coincides with that of (1) Myur ma dpa' mo (Turā-vīrā) of the Sūryagupta tradition. On the lotus petals of the inner four-petalled lotus the first four of the twenty-one types of Tārā—(2) dByaṅs can ma (east), (3) bSod nams mchog ster ma (south), (4) gTsug tor rnam rgyal ma (west) and (5) Rig byed ma (north)—are arranged. However, the *Abhisamayamuktāmālā* has modified the iconography of several Tārās of the Sūryagupta tradition.

65. Nine-deity maṇḍala of four-armed Mahākāla

Pattern: 12. Eight-spoked wheel;
Colour scheme:
Highest Yoga tantras
centred on Akṣobhya

AMM: No. 108

The last maṇḍala, which concludes the *Abhisamayamuktāmālā* and the Hahn Foundation handscroll, is the maṇḍala of four-armed Mahākāla. It seems that Mitrayogin intended to seal his maṇḍala collection with a maṇḍala of Mahākāla, the most powerful protector of Buddhism. It takes the form of an eight-spoked wheel, on the hub of which four-armed Mahākāla is depicted. According to the *Abhisamayamuktāmālā*, eight *bya rog ma* (crow-headed women) are arranged on the spokes in the eight directions, but the names of these *ḍākinī*s are not given. The Hahn Foundation possesses another coloured thangka of four-armed Mahākāla in which the eight attendants of this maṇḍala also have the heads of animals. The Ṅor maṇḍalas include another maṇḍala of Mahākāla (No. 128), but the arrangement of the attendant deities differs. The colour scheme of the courtyard is that of the Highest Yoga tantras centred on Akṣobhya (Type E).

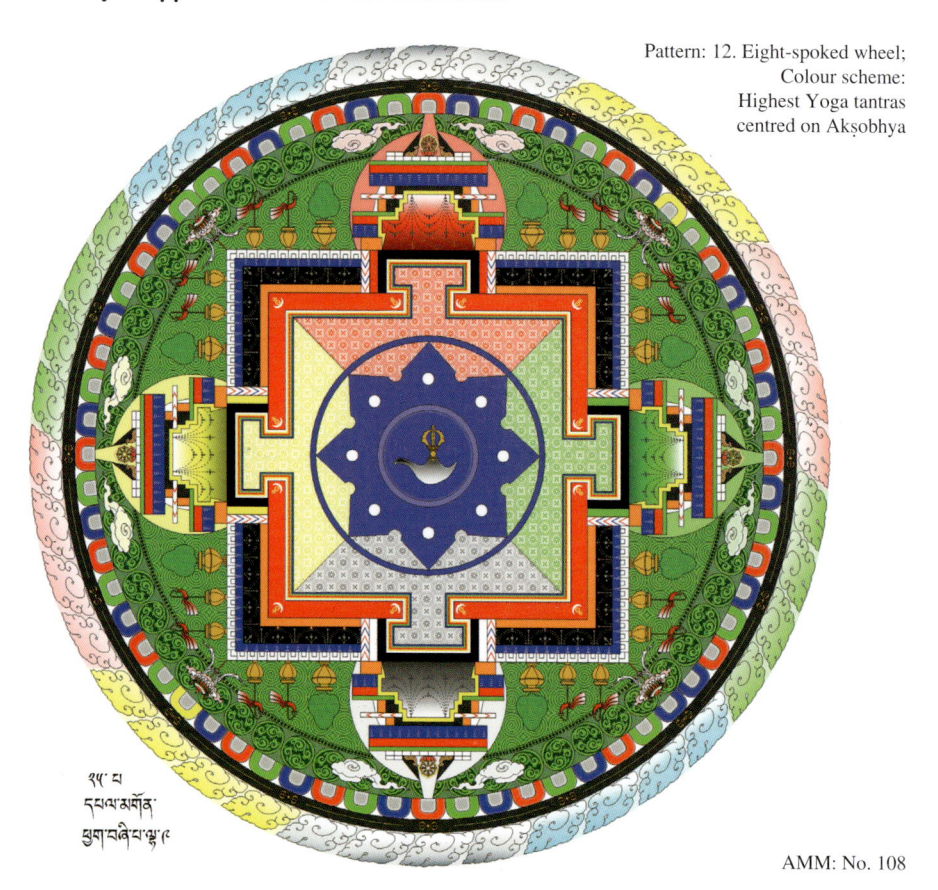

Selected Bibliography

1. Textual Sources

Lokesh Chandra. *Vajrāvalī*. Śatapiṭaka, Vol. 239. New Delhi, 1977.

Mori, Masahide 森雅秀. *The Vajrāvalī of Abhayākaragupta: Edition of Sanskrit and Tibetan Versions*. Tring, 2009.

Bhattacharyya, B. *Niṣpannayogāvalī*. Baroda, 1972.

Lee, Yonghyun 李龍賢. *The Niṣpannayogāvalī by Abhayākaragupta*. Seoul, 2003.

China Tibetology Research Center. *Patraratnamālā*. bsTan 'gyur (Danzhuer 丹珠爾), Vol. 47, pp. 963–968. Beijing, 1999.

———. *Abhisamayamuktāmālā*. Ibid., pp. 969–1079.

Roṅ tha Blo bzaṅ dam chos rgya mtsho. *rDor phreṅ daṅ mi tra sogs dkyil chog rnams las 'byuṅ ba'i yi dam rgyud sde bźi yi dkyil 'khor so so'i naṅ thig mi 'dra ba'i khyad par bźad pa bzo rig mdzes pa'i kha rgyan*. Delhi, 1978.

Tsewang Taru. *Mi tra daṅ rdor phreṅ gi lha tshogs kyi gtso bo'i sku brñan mthoṅ ba don ldan*. Delhi, 1985.

2. Hahn Foundation Handscrolls

Tanaka, Kimiaki 田中公明. *Art of Thangka* (Korean/English), Vol. 2. Seoul, 1999.

———. *Art of Thangka* (Japanese/English), Vol. 2. Kyoto, 2000.

Blurton, Richard, and Tanaka Kimiaki. *Tibetan Legacy*. Seoul, 2003.

3. General Studies on the Indo-Tibetan Maṇḍala

Tanaka, Kimiaki. *Indo-Chibetto mandara no kenkyū* インド・チベット曼荼羅の研究 [Studies in the Indo-Tibetan Maṇḍala] (in Japanese with English chapter summaries). Kyoto, 1996.

———. *Indo ni okeru mandara no seiritsu to hatten* インドにおける曼荼羅の成立と発展 [Genesis and Development of the Maṇḍala in India] (in Japanese with English summary). Tokyo, 2010.

4. Studies of the *Vajrāvalī* and *Mitra brgya rtsa* Sets of Maṇḍalas

Tanaka, Kimiaki. "How to Preserve Iconography: An Image Database of Maṇḍalas Using Computer Graphics." In *Buddhism and the 21st Century*. New Delhi, 2007.

———. "Mitrayogin's Collection of One Hundred Maṇḍalas and Their Iconography: A Handscroll in the Hahn Cultural Foundation." In *Esoteric Buddhist Studies: Identity in Diversity*. Kōyasan, 2008.

Mori, Masahide. "The Vajrāvalī Maṇḍala Series in Tibet." In *Esoteric Buddhist Studies: Identity in Diversity*. Kōyasan, 2008.

———. *Chibetto no Bukkyō bijutsu to mandara* チベットの仏教美術とマンダラ [Buddhist Art and Maṇḍalas of Tibet] (in Japanese). Nagoya, 2011.

Index of Maṇḍalas

Acala-maṇḍala (eleven-deity) (M-12) 75
Akṣobhya-maṇḍala (thirteen-deity) (M-21) 76, 84
Amoghapāśa-maṇḍala (five-deity) (M-9) 65, 72
Amṛtakuṇḍalin-maṇḍala (thirteen-deity) (V-30) 47
Aparimitāyus-maṇḍala (thirteen-deity) (M-24) 9, 87, 88

Bhairava-maṇḍala, two-armed (nine-deity) (M-45) 108
Bhairava-maṇḍala (eighteen-deity) (M-44) 107, 108
Bhūtaḍāmara-maṇḍala (thirty-four-deity) (V-40) 57
Buddhakapāla-maṇḍala (nine-deity) (V-32) 10, 49
Buddhakapāla-maṇḍala (twenty-five-deity) (V-31) 48, 49

Cakrasaṃvara-maṇḍala (thirteen-deity) (M-48) 111, 115
Cakrasaṃvara-maṇḍala (sixty-two-deity) (V-19) 8, 35, 36, 37, 38, 39, 40, 41, 48, 111, 113, 121
Chinnamastakā-Vārāhī-maṇḍala (thirteen-deity) (M-55) 118
Citta-Hevajra-maṇḍala (nine-deity) (V-6) 23
Citta-Hevajra-maṇḍala (seventeen-deity) (V-15) 32, 33, 34

Ḍākinī-maṇḍala (nine-deity, as transmitted by Maitrīpa) (M-57) 120
Dharmadhātuvāgīśvara-maṇḍala (V-39) 7, 12, 56, 100

Garbha-Hevajra-maṇḍala (nine-deity) (V-5) 22
Garbha-Hevajra-maṇḍala (seventeen-deity) (V-14) 31, 32
Garuḍa-Vajrapāṇi-maṇḍala (five-deity) (M-19) 82
Grahamātṛkā-maṇḍala (twenty-one-deity) (V-44) 61
Guhyasamāja-Akṣobhyavajra-maṇḍala (thirty-two-deity) (V-2) 19
Guhyasamāja-Mañjuvajra-maṇḍala (nineteen-deity) 7, 18

Hayagrīva-maṇḍala (seventeen-deity) (M-11) 74, 75
Hayagrīva-Padmanarteśvara-maṇḍala (eighteen-deity) (M-63) 10, 126

Jambhala-maṇḍala (nine-deity) (M-5) 68, 69
Jinasāgara-maṇḍala (thirteen-deity) (M-62) 125
Jñānaḍākinī-maṇḍala (thirteen-deity) (V-35) 10, 52

Kāya-Hevajra-maṇḍala (nine-deity) (V-8) 25
Kāya-Hevajra-maṇḍala (seventeen-deity) (V-17) 34
Kāyavākcittapariniṣpanna-Kālacakra-maṇḍala (V-36) 8, 12, 53

Krodhahūṃkāra-maṇḍala (eleven-deity) (V-25) 42
Kṛṣṇayamāri-maṇḍala (thirteen-deity) (V-4) 21
Kurukullā-maṇḍala (fifteen-deity) (V-12) 29

Mahācakravajrapāṇi-maṇḍala (fourteen-deity) (M-46) 109
Mahākāla-maṇḍala, four-armed (nine-deity) (M-65) 7, 128
Mahākāruṇika-maṇḍala (thirteen-deity) (M-8) 9, 71, 84
Mahāmāyā-maṇḍala (five-deity, small) (M-61) 124
Mahāmāyā-maṇḍala (five-deity, medium) (M-60) 123
Mahāmāyā-maṇḍala (six-deity) (V-33) 50, 124
Mañjughoṣa-maṇḍala, white (five-deity) (M-7) 70
Mañjughoṣa-maṇḍala (seventeen-deity, as transmitted by Candragomin) (M-36) 99
Mañjughoṣa-maṇḍala (twenty-one-deity, profound tradition) (M-37) 100
Mañjughoṣa-maṇḍala (fifty-three-deity, as transmitted by Vilāsavajra) (M-35) 98
Mārīcī-maṇḍala (twenty-five-deity) (V-41) 58

Nairātmyā-maṇḍala (fifteen-deity) (V-11) 28, 29
Nairātmyā-maṇḍala (twenty-three-deity) (V-10) 27, 28
Navoṣṇīṣa-maṇḍala (thirty-seven-deity) (V-38) 55, 87
Nīlāmbaradharavajrapāṇi-maṇḍala (single-deity) (M-16) 79

One hundred clans maṇḍala (one-hundred-deity) (M-39) 102

Pañcaḍāka-maṇḍala (V-9) 8, 12, 26
Pañcarakṣā-maṇḍala (thirteen-deity) (V-42) 10, 59
Paramādya-Vajrasattva-maṇḍala (sixty-one-deity) (M-34) 10, 97
Parṇaśavarī-maṇḍala (five-deity) (M-2) 65
Prajñāpāramitā-maṇḍala (sixty-four-deity) (M-38) 101

Raktayamāri-maṇḍala (thirteen-deity) (M-42) 105

Sahajasaṃvara-maṇḍala (five-deity) (M-49) 112
Śākyamuni-maṇḍala (thirty-five-deity) (M-6) 10, 69
Saṃvara-maṇḍala (eight-deity, as transmitted by Advayavajra) (M-51) 114
Saṃvara-maṇḍala (nine-deity, as transmitted by Tilopa) (M-50) 113
Saṃvara-maṇḍala, two-armed (sixty-two-deity) (V-20) 37, 38
Saṃvara-maṇḍala, white (twenty-nine-deity) (M-47) 110, 121
Saṃvara-maṇḍala, yellow (sixty-two-deity) (V-21) 38, 41
Saṃvara-Vajrasattva-maṇḍala (thirty-seven-deity) (V-18) 35
Sarasvatī-maṇḍala (thirteen-deity) (M-1) 7, 64
Sarvajagadvinaya-maṇḍala (fifty-seven-deity) (M-33) 96
Sarvārthasiddhi-maṇḍala (fifty-seven-deity) (M-32) 95
Sarvārthasiddhi-Vārāhī-maṇḍala (thirteen-deity) (M-54) 117
Sarvavid-Vairocana-maṇḍala (one-hundred-and-five-deity) (M-23) 86, 87, 102
Ṣaṭcakravartin-maṇḍala (V-26) 8, 12, 43
Siṃhanāda-maṇḍala (five-deity) (M-10) 73
Sitātapatrā-maṇḍala (twenty-nine-deity) (M-3) 66

Tārā-maṇḍala (twenty-one types of, as transmitted by Sūryagupta) (M-64) 127
Trailokyavijaya-maṇḍala (fifty-seven-deity) (M-31) 94, 95, 96

Uṣṇīṣavijayā-maṇḍala (nine-deity) (M-4) 62, 66, 67
Uṣṇīṣavijayā-maṇḍala (thirty-three-deity) (V-45) 7, 62

Vairocana-Mañjuvajra-maṇḍala (forty-three-deity) (V-3) 10, 20
Vajrabhairava-maṇḍala (nine-deity) (M-43) 106
Vajradhātu-maṇḍala (fifty-three-deity) (V-37) 8, 20, 54, 64, 94
Vajragaruḍa-maṇḍala (nine-deity) (M-20) 83
Vajraheruka-maṇḍala (twenty-one-deity) (V-29) 46
Vajrahūṃkāra-maṇḍala (twenty-nine-deity) (V-28) 45
Vajrajvālānalārka-maṇḍala (seventeen-deity) (M-27) 90
Vajrāmṛta-maṇḍala (twenty-one-deity) (V-27) 44, 46, 47
Vajrapāṇi-maṇḍala (single-deity) (M-15) 78
Vajrapāṇi-maṇḍala (five-stūpa) (M-17) 80
Vajrapāṇi-maṇḍala (nine-deity) (M-14) 77
Vajrapāṇi-maṇḍala (thirteen-deity) (M-18) 81
Vajrapāṇi-maṇḍala (thirteen-deity) (M-25) 88
Vajrapāṇi-maṇḍala, surrounded by the eight great *nāga*s (thirteen-deity) (M-30) 93
Vajrapāṇi-maṇḍala (seventeen-deity, as transmitted by Sugatigarbha) (M-22) 85
Vajrapāṇi-maṇḍala, surrounded by the protectors of the ten directions and the four great kings (twenty-three-deity) (M-28) 91
Vajrapāṇi-maṇḍala (forty-five-deity) (M-29) 92
Vajrapāṇicakravartin-maṇḍala (one-hundred-and-thirty-eight-deity) (M-26) 89
Vajrasattva-maṇḍala (seventeen-deity) (M-40) 103
Vajratārā-maṇḍala (nineteen-deity) (V-13) 30
Vajravārāhī-maṇḍala, three-headed and six-armed (thirteen-deity) (M-52) 115
Vajravārāhī-maṇḍala, two-headed (thirteen-deity) (M-53) 116
Vajravārāhī-maṇḍala, red (thirty-seven-deity) (V-22) 39, 40, 41
Vajravārāhī-maṇḍala, blue (thirty-seven-deity) (V-23) 40
Vajravārāhī-maṇḍala, yellow (thirty-seven-deity) (V-24) 41
Vajravidāraṇa-maṇḍala (twenty-three-deity) (M-13) 76
Vāk-Hevajra-maṇḍala (nine-deity) (V-7) 24
Vāk-Hevajra-maṇḍala (seventeen-deity) (V-16) 33
Vārāhī-maṇḍala (thirteen-deity, as transmitted by Nāropa) (M-56) 119
Vārāhī-maṇḍala, black and four-headed (five-deity) (M-59) 122
Vārāhī-maṇḍala (thirty-seven-deity) (M-58) 121
Vasudhārā-maṇḍala (nineteen-deity) (V-43) 60

Yamāntaka-maṇḍala, six-headed (twenty-one-deity) (M-41) 104
Yogāmbara-maṇḍala (fifty-eight-deity) (V-34) 51

On the Hahn Cultural Foundation, Seoul

The Hahn Cultural Foundation, the owner of the original scrolls of the CG maṇḍalas, was founded by Dr. Hahn Kwang-ho (CBE), who established many medical and chemical companies in Korea. Developing an early interest in and appreciation of fine art and antiques, he has collected artworks from Korea and around the world over the past fifty years. In particular, he became fascinated with Tibetan art after purchasing some Tibetan thangkas in London where he happened to visit on business. His collection has been growing yearly and has reached as many as 2,500 items. It is now the largest collection of Tibetan art in the world. In 1996, on the recommendation of the late Prof. Namio Egami, this author was asked to compile the official catalogue of the Tibetan paintings in the possession of the foundation. Since then, six volumes of the "Art of Thangka" series have been published.

In September 1999, the Hwa-jeong Museum, which is run by the foundation, was opened to the public in Itaewon, Seoul, and the exhibition "Art of Tibet" was held to commemorate its opening. In 2001–2002, "The World of Thangka" exhibition was circulated in five museums in

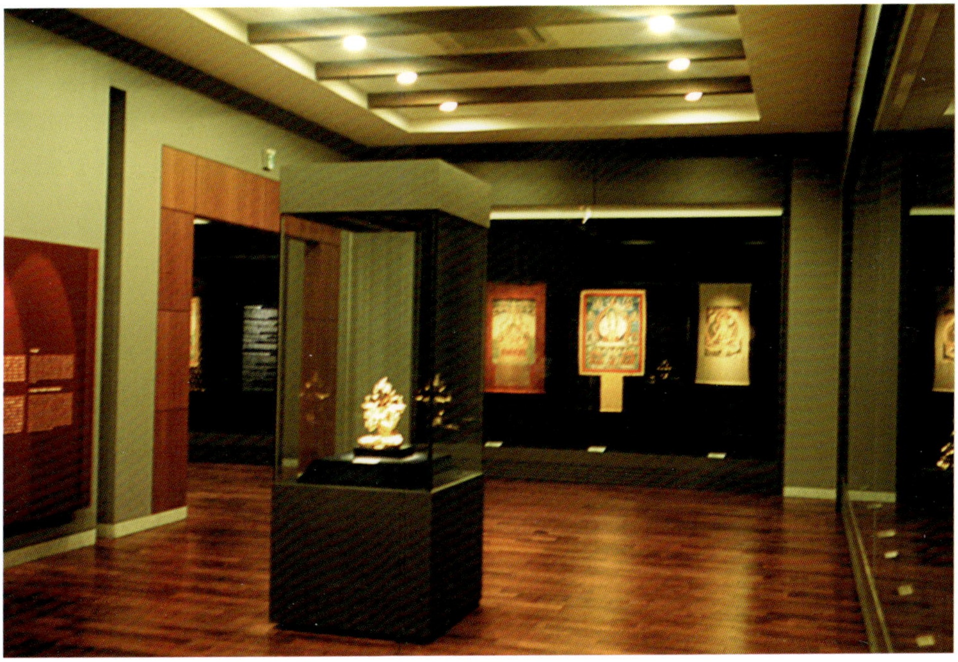

Japan with 53,000 attendees in total. In addition, the "Tibetan Legacy" exhibition was held at the British Museum in September 2003.

The foundation has thus been active in organizing exhibitions. However, the former Hwa-jeong Musuem was too small to exhibit and store such a large collection. The foundation began the construction of a new four-storeyed museum equipped with large storage space in Pyeongchang-dong, Seoul, and opened it to the public in May 2006. The Tibetan collection occupies the first floor of the museum, and the other floors are used for other collections and temporary exhibitions. The original handscrolls that are the subject of the present book are not always exhibited. For details of exhibitions, contact:

273-1, Pyeongchang-Dong, Jongno-Gu, Seoul, 110-012, Korea
Tel: +82-2-2075-0114; Fax: +82-2-2075-0130
E-mail: hahnbit@chol.com
http://www.hjmuseum.org

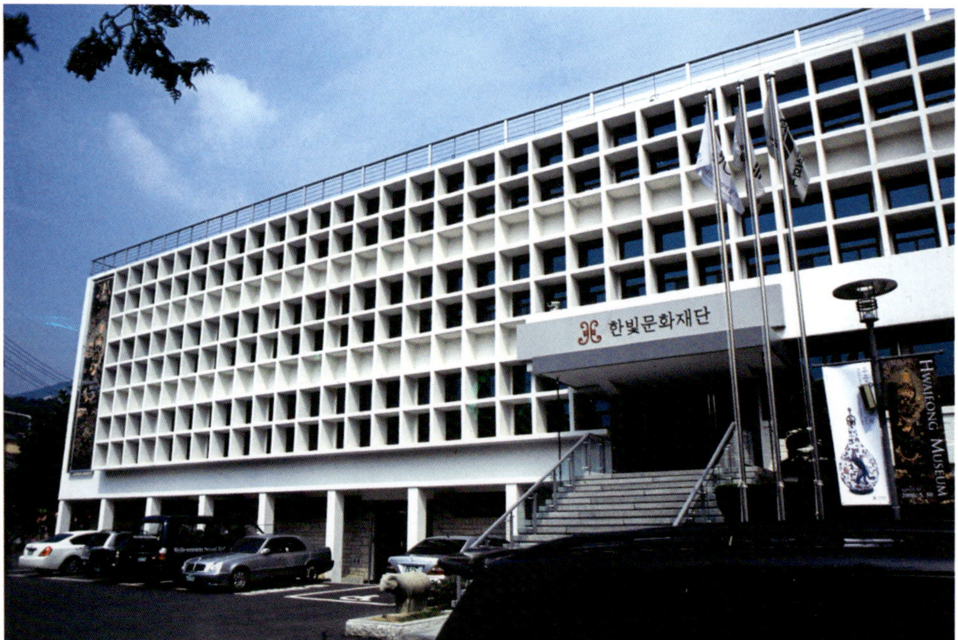

Toga Meditation Museum

Toga Meditation Museum (Meisō no Sato) is a unique theme park focusing on Tibeto-Nepalese Buddhist art that was established by a local government body in Toyama prefecture, Japan. The museum is now managed by a quasi-public corporation named Toga Furusato Foundation. The main exhibits in the Meditation Museum are six Buddhist paintings: the one hundred peaceful and wrathful deities, Amitābha and his Pure Land, One-thousand-armed Avalokiteśvara, the Garbha-maṇḍala, and the Vajradhātu-maṇḍala, each measuring 4 by 4 metres. They were painted in Toga by Mr. Sashi Dhoj Tulachan, a Thakali Buddhist painter from Toga's sister village, Tukuche in lower Mustang, Nepal. After the completion of the paintings, the village constructed a museum to enshrine them. The village then added a restaurant, a guesthouse, and a beautiful garden in the shape of a maṇḍala.

The author has participated in the project since the painter's first visit to Toga in 1989, and he was appointed chief curator of the museum in 1997. In July 2006, the CG maṇḍalas of the *Vajrāvalī* and *Mitra brgya rtsa* sets were opened to the public as permanent exhibits. The museum is open daily except on Wednesdays and is closed during the winter (December–March) since it is located in an area with heavy snowfall.

Tibet Culture Centre International

The Tibet Culture Centre was established in 1972 to introduce and provide correct information about Tibetan culture to the Japanese public on a membership basis. As of January 2010, the President of the Association is Ryūzō Takayama (ex-professor of Osaka Industrial University), and the Managing Director is Pema Gyalpo (professor at Tōin Yokohama University). The main aim of this Culture Centre is to assist and encourage the development of all Tibetan culture in the fields of religion, arts, language, history, and customs through ethnological as well as anthropological research and to encourage the Japanese public to gain an understanding of Tibet. To achieve this aim, regular classes are conducted on Buddhism, culture, arts, and language by native Tibetan teachers. The author has been Vice-President of the Association since January 2009 and a lecturer on Indo-Tibetan Buddhism since 2006, in conjunction with his work at the Nakamura Hajime Eastern Institute, his principal place of employment. For further information, contact: http: //www16.ocn.ne.jp/~tcc/

Dr. Kimiaki TANAKA (b. 1955, Fukuoka) studied Indian Philosophy and Sanskrit Philology at the University of Tokyo, completing a doctoral thesis entitled "Genesis and Development of the Maṇḍala in India."

He has been lecturer at the University of Tokyo and Takushoku University, teaching Tibetan as well as courses on Buddhism, and held a Spalding Visiting Fellowship at Oxford University (Wolfson College) in 1993. As a visiting professor, he gave lectures on Sino-Japanese cultural exchange at Beijing Centre for Japanese Studies in 2003 and 2010.

He is presently a research fellow of the Nakamura Hajime Eastern Institute and a lecturer in art history (Buddhist Iconography) at Keio University, Tokyo. He is also chief curator of the Toga Meditation Museum in Toyama prefecture, Vice-President of the Tibet Culture Centre International in Tokyo and Academic Consultant to the Hahn Cultural Foundation in Seoul.

He has published 30 books and 90 articles on Esoteric Buddhism, Buddhist iconography and Tibetan art. For further details, contact: http://www.geocities.jp/dkyil_hkhor/

The author and the publisher, Mr. Bidur Dangol

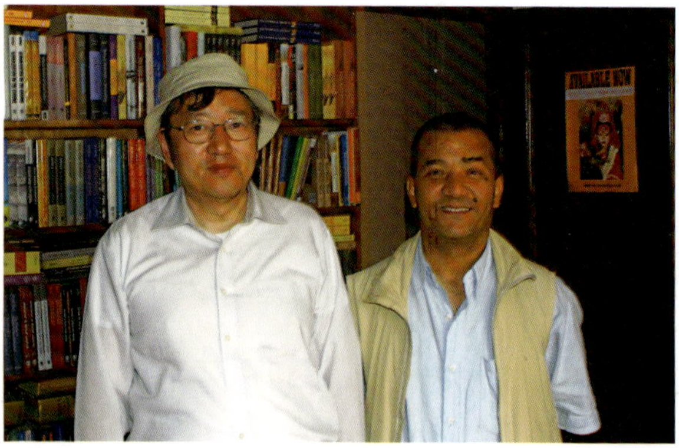